MICRO-ENTERPRISE AND PERSONALISATION

What size is good care?

Catherine Needham, Kerry Allen and Kelly Hall

First published in Great Britain in 2017 by

Policy Press
University of Bristol
1-9 Old Park Hill
Bristol
BS2 8BB
UK
t: +44 (0)117 954 5940
pp-info@bristol.ac.uk
www.policypress.co.uk

North America office:
Policy Press
c/o The University of Chicago Press
1427 East 60th Street
Chicago, IL 60637, USA
t: +1 773 702 7700
f: +1 773-702-9756
sales@press.uchicago.edu
www.press.uchicago.edu

© Policy Press 2017

British Library Cataloguing in Publication Data
A catalogue record for this book is available from the British Library

Library of Congress Cataloging-in-Publication Data
A catalog record for this book has been requested

ISBN 978-1-4473-1922-1 hardcover
ISBN 978-1-4473-1923-8 paperback
ISBN 978-1-4473-1926-9 ePub
ISBN 978-1-4473-1927-6 Mobi
ISBN 978-1-4473-1924-5 ePDF

Cover design by Andrew Corbett
Front cover: image kindly supplied by Getty
Printed and bound in Great Britain by CPI Group (UK) Ltd,
Croydon, CR0 4YY
Policy Press uses environmentally responsible print partners

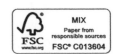

Contents

List of figures, tables and boxes

Figures

Tables

Boxes

Acknowledgements

This book has been a long time in the making and has drawn on the insight, experience and expertise of a wide range of people. The journey from a 2011 research grant application to the Economic and Social Research Council (ESRC) to a 2016 book has involved a lot of talking, thinking and reflecting about organisational size and about what makes for good-quality care and support.

We would like to thank the ESRC, whose funding of the research – as a project entitled Does Smaller mean Better? Evaluating Micro-enterprises in Adult Social Care (ESRC Standard Grant ES/K002317/1) – made everything else possible.

We would also like to thank our colleagues at the University of Birmingham, and beyond. Stephen McKay (University of Lincoln) undertook quantitative and financial data analysis. Jon Glasby (University of Birmingham) advised on project design, data analysis and evaluation. Sarah Carr (Middlesex University) contributed to the literature review. Rosemary Littlechild and Denise Tanner (University of Birmingham) evaluated the co-researcher involvement. At regular project team meetings, all of these people challenged our thinking and helped steer the path of the research. Many other colleagues looked at draft chapters and provided very helpful comments on our work.

People who use services and carers were involved as co-researchers on the project, contributing to the design of interview materials, leading interviews, assisting in data analysis and helping to disseminate the findings. Their involvement enriched the research process in so many ways, generating insights that would not have been possible without them, as well as keeping us focused on making research meaningful beyond an academic audience. The co-researchers were Tracey Bealey, Isabelle Brant, Hayley Broxup, Roy Doré, Peggy Dunne, Sandra Harris, John Kerry, Simon MacGregor, Adrian Murray, Joan Rees, Anna Stevenson, Brian Timmins, David Walker, Joanne Ward, Gareth Welford and Sheila Wharton. We hope to find ways to work together again.

Many organisations helped us gain access to research sites or to communicate the findings in a range of ways. Community Catalysts and their local coordinators helped connect us to micro-enterprises. Local authorities in the three localities in which we did the research helped to facilitate links to local social care providers. The Social Care Institute for Excellence (SCIE) gave support on communications.

Laura Brodrick from Think Big Picture provided graphic illustration of events and created rich pictures which further stimulated our thinking.

We would like to extend particular thanks to the case study organisations themselves and to the individuals and families using their services, who generously gave up their time to be interviewed. Research would be impossible without the willingness of people to allow researchers into their homes and offices, and we are perpetually surprised and grateful that people agree so readily to being interviewed.

Finally, we would like to thank our families for allowing us to commit time to a book project, which never quite fitted into the working day.

List of abbreviations

ASCOT	Adult Social Care Outcomes Toolkit
BME	black and minority ethnic
CIC	Community Interest Company
CQC	Care Quality Commission
DH	Department of Health
FTE	full-time equivalent
LGBT	lesbian, gay, bisexual and transgender
NAAPS	National Association of Adult Placement Schemes
NAVCA	National Association for Voluntary and Community Action
NHS	National Health Service
NPM	new public management
PA	personal assistant
SCIE	Social Care Institute for Excellence
SCRQoL	social care-related quality of life
TLAP	Think Local, Act Personal

ONE

Introduction: what size is 'just right' for a care provider?

As public service providers strive to improve, a common concern is to ensure that they are operating at an optimal size. Hospitals merge with others to achieve economies of scale. Schools that are perceived to be underperforming federate with more successful neighbours to share management teams. Within the social care sector, care homes link up with others in national chains to reduce costs and increase clout in tendering processes. While these examples demonstrate the perceived advantages of expansion, there are also examples of public services reducing their scale to become better fit for purpose. Social work teams spin out of local authorities to form small mutuals that aim to focus better on the core role. Charities split part of their work into a social enterprise that can operate with more flexible financing. Patterns of preferred sizing may depend on the function of the organisation, but they may also be cyclical over time, shifting from 'big is efficient' to 'small is responsive' and back again (Pollitt, 2008). Governments often send ambivalent signals about what size of service provider is preferred: small community social enterprises are encouraged at the same time as larger tendering processes reward consortia of providers (McCabe and Phillimore, 2012).

Understanding better the relationship between the size and performance of public service providers is a key element of service improvement, and this book tests that relationship in the distinctive context of care. Organisational size and performance of public service providers has been examined as part of broader studies of public management (for a meta-analysis see Boyne, 2003a). However, much of this literature relates to education and health, or to US welfare studies with limited applicability outside that national context. Writing about the closely related issue of scale, Postma notes, 'Empirical studies that take scale seriously as an object of study in itself are lacking … Because of the high expectations and the frequent use of (changes in) scale as a governance instrument, empirical studies of the workings of scale in practice are necessary' (Postma, 2015, pp 23, 25).

This book picks up Postma's challenge, taking size (and scale) seriously as an object of study and focusing particularly on the size of organisations delivering social care. It does so by considering the contribution that micro-enterprises (employing five people or fewer) can make to the care sector, by comparing them to larger care providers. The personalisation agenda in social care creates an environment in which organisations are being asked to work at a human scale, delivering person-centred support rather than standardised 'time and task' approaches to care (Needham, 2011). However, much of the literature on personalisation has been normative, and based on vignettes of individual experience – what Beresford (2008, p 17) calls 'cosy stories of a few people's gains'. What we provide here is a theoretically informed and rigorous mixed-methods approach to understand better the contribution that small-scale care services make to the delivery of this policy agenda. The large scale of our work (interviewing almost 150 people) is unprecedented in comparative studies of care organisations. Ours is also the first study to compare the costs and outcomes of micro-enterprise with those of larger organisations, combining qualitative interviewing with a validated outcome measure (the Adult Social Care Outcomes Toolkit (ASCOT)). We have undertaken this approach alongside co-researchers who have experience of using care services or of caring for someone who uses these services. Through these aspects of our approach we are able to address significant policy and practice questions at a time when sustained austerity makes such questions ever more crucial. We also contribute to academic debates about the relationship between organisational size, performance and innovation, and how best to operationalise these as research variables while also recognising their socially constructed and performative dimensions.

From macro to micro

Fashions in the size of public service organisations come and go, and proceed in differently paced cycles in different countries. The country focus of this book is England, where the previous twenty years can be characterised as periods in which health and social care services have proceeded in the direction of larger organisational forms. The care management reforms in social care in the early 1990s, which facilitated the outsourcing of many care services to the private and third sectors, have over time led to a dominance of large private sector providers, offering domiciliary care (help at home with washing, dressing and food preparation) or residential care (Gray and Birrell, 2013). In health, hospitals have merged into foundation trusts spread over several sites, and trusts are forming partnerships with shared leadership teams (NHS

England, 2015). GPs' practices are increasingly merging into large, multi-site practices (Smith et al, 2013).

In the National Health Service (NHS) these trends continue to gather momentum whereas, in social care there has been more soul searching about the quality and sustainability of large-scale care services (Public Accounts Committee, 2011; CQC, 2015; Skills for Care, 2015). The concurrent policy agendas of personalisation, austerity and localism are leading policy makers to promote the benefits of using small, community-based organisations more extensively in the delivery of care services. Personalisation has led to more people being given control over their own care spend as a 'personal budget', with a promise that they can then purchase services that more closely meet their individual preferences (Putting People First, 2007). Making this individualised commissioning a reality requires a diverse range of options for people, and information and support to use that choice effectively. The Care Act 2014 affirms the importance of market development if personalisation is to be meaningful for people. Local authorities now have a duty to ensure that people within the social care system – frail older people, disabled people and people accessing mental health services – can have choice and control over the people who support them. The Care Act also makes clear that local authorities have a duty to ensure that self-funders – those with assets that push them above the means-test threshold for state funding – have access to a diverse range of options.

This context creates a demand for local diversity that very small community-based organisations could help to satisfy. As a Department of Health (DH) guidance document asserts, 'Micro social care and support enterprises established and managed by local people are in a good position to deliver individualised services and are vital elements of a diverse market' (DH, 2010). Very small organisations seem to offer an intuitive fit with individualised commissioning by a personal budget holder. These micro-providers can be 'close to the user' in a spatial sense, by being located in the same communities, and also in an interpersonal sense, if very small providers can develop closer relationships with the people being supported (Needham, 2015).

However, the evidence base for the benefits of micro care provision is limited. There are lots of positive case studies put forward by the micro-enterprise support organisation Community Catalysts, and many of these have featured in publications from the DH and the social care sector umbrella body Think Local, Act Personal (TLAP) (DH and NAAPS, 2009; Community Catalysts, 2011, 2014; TLAP, 2011). Some of these examples are particularly striking because they differ from the norm of social care provision – particularly for older people's care in the home – which is dominated by a model of short visits several times a day to do highly specified tasks (Burstow, 2014). Micro-enterprise examples such as a fishing group for older men with dementia, or a dance class run by and for people with learning disabilities, constitute a very different offer. However, it is hard to assess from these good-news stories the extent to which they are isolated examples of a different way of working, or early signs of system change in social care.

The preference for individual case studies is also apparent in the broader literature on small business: detailed case studies are common, but it is hard to use these to understand the 'complex ways in which the small scale sector is integrated into the economy' (Curran, 1990, p 139, cited in Edwards and Ram, 2006, p 896). Edwards and Ram (2006, p 900) argue that, outside of individual case studies, small business research relies on surveys that lack contextual detail; instead they call for studies that sit between these two extremes. It is into this space – between individual organisational case studies and large-scale surveys – that our research makes its distinctive contribution as a study that gathers outcome data and qualitative interview material from 143 people in 27 organisations in order to build the evidence base surrounding micro-enterprises within social care. We take the policy claims that are made about micro-enterprises as hypotheses, which are tested against qualitative and quantitative research findings from people who use and provide services across a range of different-size categories. In particular we focus on four claims that are made by proponents of micro forms of service delivery: that micro-enterprises are more personalised, innovative, cost-effective and outcomes oriented than larger organisations (Putting People First, 2007; DH, 2010; NAAPS, 2010; NHS Foundation, 2011).

To evaluate these four claims we undertook primary research in three areas of England, sampled to differ from each other in their regional and demographic profiles. The three case study localities we chose were a metropolitan borough council in the North West of England, a mixed urban, suburban and rural setting across two boroughs in the West Midlands, and a county in the East Midlands. The sites were selected (a) to differ from each other in their regional profiles (urban, suburban and rural) and demography (variance in levels of affluence and age of population) and (b) on advice from project partners about areas with a known network of micro-enterprises, to overcome issues related to the low visibility of such organisations (Phillimore et al, 2009).

We are aware that the commitment to person-centred care services, individualised budgets and more diverse markets of providers is not limited to England and that some of the impetus for personalised approaches in the UK came from broader international trends (Izuhara, 2003; Carr and Robbins, 2009; Glasby and Dickinson, 2009; Grit and de Bont, 2010; Land and Himmelweit, 2010). However, there is enormous diversity in the practical application of these care arrangements between countries, which hampers the like-for-like comparisons we required so as to understand better the implications of different sizes of care provider. We aimed to keep the national policy context of personalisation as stable as possible to assist generalisation. Within the UK, we limited our research to England because of the increased difficulty of generalising across the four component parts of the United Kingdom, particularly in relation to social care services (Gray and Birrell, 2013). England, Scotland, Wales and Northern Ireland are all moving at different speeds towards person-centred care services, and the commitment to market diversity that is embedded in England's Care Act 2014 is not so evident in other parts of the UK (Gray and Birrell, 2013; Pearson et al, 2014).

The research focused on 27 organisations of different sizes that provide care and support – nine in each of the three localities. We interviewed staff and people who use the service, or who care for someone who uses it. We focused the research on organisations supporting older people and/or adults with learning disabilities to provide diversity within the cases, while avoiding stretching the focus too thinly across a range of different types of people who are eligible for social care services. It enabled comparison between groups with different profiles: for example, young adults with disabilities tend to receive larger care packages and to have had access to personalised approaches over a longer time frame than older people. People with experience of local care services were involved as co-researchers, engaged in research design, interviewing, analysis and dissemination.

The scope of the research – 27 organisations, 143 interviews – is broad for a mainly qualitative study, although we are aware it is not large enough to make claims about statistical generalisability. We suggest that our findings are generalisable to theory in the way that Popay et al set out: 'the aim is to make logical generalizations to a theoretical understanding of a similar class of phenomena rather than probabilistic generalizations to a population'. Our analysis of micro-enterprises allows for 'the generation of the logical features of a type against which further cases can be examined with gradual evolution of our theoretical understanding' (Popay et al, 1998, pp 348–9) Through analysing the research data we offer theoretical insights into the relationship between organisational size and care and contribute to theoretical understandings of performance, innovation and personalisation in a care setting.

In the chapters that follow, we present the research and its findings, and our analysis of the extent to which care services can be improved by developing more organisations that operate at a micro scale. The book also links the findings into broader debates about organisational size and performance, contributing to public management literature about what drives performance in public services. Here we set out how micro-enterprises are defined before giving more details of our approach to the research and what follows in the rest of the book.

What are micro-enterprises?

The term micro-enterprise, like social enterprise, lacks a fixed definition (MacGillivray et al, 2001; Fiedler, 2007; Pattie and Johnston, 2011). It is used within the social care sector to refer to organisations that employ five staff or fewer (full-time equivalent (FTE)) (DH, 2010). These organisations have a range of legal forms, including charities, sole traders, partnerships, community interest companies and mutuals. Thus, they are a mixture of for-profit and not-for-profit organisations. The care sector workforce support organisation Skills for Care estimates that almost a third (31%) of registered care providers have fewer than five FTE members of staff, with almost 5,500 such organisations operating across England. Even this is likely to be an under-estimation, as it excludes sole traders and self-employed people who are not registered for VAT (Skills for Care, 2015).

Micro-enterprises are commonly set up to meet the needs of an individual or small group (Shared Lives Plus, no date). Some are set up by front-line staff previously based in large organisations, whereas others are created by people who need support or by carers. These micro-enterprises may provide core 'care' services (such as day support services; domiciliary care; residential care), or may have a broader focus (such as leisure, therapies, employment) (DH, 2010).

Micro-enterprises in the care sector vary widely from each other. While five FTE staff is the threshold, some micro-providers employ ten or more staff on a part-time basis. Others are sole traders, working on their own. Examples of some of the micro-enterprises that were included in the research are given in Box 1.1, along with indications of what their owners consider to be their distinctive contribution. They are separated out into the four different types of care provision that we encountered in the sector, discussed more in Chapter Five. Names are changed here and elsewhere in the book to preserve anonymity.

Box 1.1: Examples of micro-enterprises

Micro domiciliary care service

Full Lives was set up by Janet, who previously worked within local authority care services and wanted the opportunity to run her own support service. It now has four members of staff, supporting three people. The work varies between personal care in the home, and support to access activities outside the home. Janet says, "Because we are a small company we can be more flexible, at the hours people want. We don't have a lot of clients so we get to know the people we work with. You can build up strong relationships."

Micro day support

Pam runs a day service with six part-time staff. She feels that the small size allows them to support the social integration of people with learning disabilities, including Pam's daughter. Pam explains: "I set up Woodlands because day centres were closing ... and there wasn't anything [else]." Woodlands is based in a semi-rural community and aims to connect people to the community: "our members go out and get recognised by the shopkeepers and people and they develop relationships with folks in the community", says Pam.

Micro accommodation

Our House is a micro-enterprise providing shared accommodation to men with learning disabilities. The owner provides low-level support beyond the landlord role, including social support and activities. As one tenant explains: "He does things out of his way to get you out the house. He'll ... come round once a week and just check in with us ... and he's very protective as well, because say if you wanted a mobile contract ... he goes 'right, well give me about two days, I'll look it up', he'll come back with a better deal."

Micro one-to-one support

Barbara works on her own, providing help in the home to 14 people in her local area. The support she provides is very diverse, from preparing food to cleaning out cupboards and taking people to the doctor's or to concerts. She said: "We had our redundancy [from a care agency]. I was always getting in trouble for doing too much, like cooking meals and doing somebody's washing. And when I was made redundant, that was it. I just made me mind up I was going to do it."

Finding micro-enterprises to include in a research study can be challenging, given that these organisations may not appear on local lists of preferred providers or be registered with the regulator, the Care Quality Commission (CQC). To overcome low visibility we located the research in three areas of England that had a micro-enterprise coordinator based within the local authority. We are aware that this limits the typicality of the site sample, since only a small number of local authorities will have a micro-enterprise coordinator in place. The micro-enterprise support organisation Community Catalysts, which supports the coordinator model, has worked with around 10% of local authorities to develop their micro care sectors. However, we felt this approach to identifying localities (a form of purposive sampling) would give us an insight into the potential for micro-enterprises to make a contribution in the context of a supportive local authority. Since all local authorities are now mandated by the Care Act to support market diversity, we saw these localities as early adopters of approaches that are becoming increasingly mainstream.

We sampled organisations from a list of local micro-enterprises given to us by the coordinator in each site. This approach means that we included only organisations that were visible to the coordinators. Other studies have investigated 'below the radar' groups that operate informally within communities, often on a voluntary basis, and are largely invisible to formal organisations like local government (Phillimore et al, 2009). In our study we were primarily interested in exploring the potential for micro-enterprises to contribute to formal care provision without the informal and ad hoc nature of much below-the-radar work, but also without the intensification associated with some large-scale care provision. This focus allowed us to examine whether micro-enterprises can be an effective alternative to existing paid-for care services where the quality as a sector has often been considered to be poor (EHRC, 2011; Lewis and West, 2014). We included only organisations that had a trading income – that is, they levy a charge for their services, which is paid by the user directly or by the local authority on their behalf. Many care and support services provided by charities and the statutory sector do not charge, but we did not include those here, so as to avoid problems of comparability between too many different types of organisation.

The approach to the research

As the study aims to have policy relevance, and was funded by a research council, we were alert to the need to undertake the research in such a way that it satisfied norms of 'hard' social science enquiry. Our investigation of the contribution of micro-enterprises to adult social care started with the formulation of a set of hypotheses that we tested through the comparison of differently sized care providers, viewed as proportionate units of study. A validated tool was used to develop quantitative outcome scores for each study participant using care service, and we analysed pricing data so as to establish a value-for-money relationship between outcome scores and service costs.

However, consistent with a critical-realist ontology, we were aware that such methods can identify patterns and establish relationships but cannot satisfactorily explain those patterns or relationships (Edwards et al, 2004). Approaches to research located in critical realism provide a framework where positivist enquiry can be deepened by abductive and interpretivist research practice to move towards 'thick explanation' (O'Mahoney and Vincent, 2014). Critical realism is an approach initiated by Bhaskar (1997; 1998) and widely developed and applied. Here in particular we drew on applications of critical realism that resonate with research design, the philosophy of social science and the nature of public service organisations, offered by Pawson and Tilley (1997), Sayer (2000), Currie et al (2010) and Edwards et al (2004).

Bhaskar (1997) acknowledged that the transitive dimension (theories and knowledge of the world) was not straightforwardly linked to the intransitive dimension (the physical natural world). This position sets the critical-realist approach apart from positivist philosophy, where the truth can be known. In Sayer's (2000) analysis, Bhaskar's distinction between what is 'real' and what is 'empirical' also sets critical realism apart from social-constructionist approaches, where all experiences have their own reality. Instead Bhaskar frames the 'real' as the mechanisms that have agency and power, that can cause an effect, whether natural or social (Sayer, 2000, p 11). This realm of the 'real' is different from what we think of as individual lived experience and perspective.

By recognising the significance of 'the real' − the causal − critical realism can be the basis for an abductive approach for social science enquiry, combining aspects of deductive and inductive reasoning (Blaikie, 2009; Schwartz-Shea and Yanow, 2012). Our approach, in line with critical realism, was to pursue deductive hypothesis testing (an understanding of how micro-enterprises perform) while acknowledging that we would not reveal one 'true' or complete picture of how different providers operate within a complex system with multiple mechanisms, many of which may remain hidden from us. As a means of assessing the extent to which outcomes are realised for individual service users, we recognise the value of standardised quantitative measures such as ASCOT, developed by the University of Kent and used by the DH in its national social care survey. Using validated tools enhances the reliability of the research and allows the findings from our study to be compared against those of others. Such tools also have a currency in the policy world, and we were keen that our research would be useful for and used by policy makers and practitioners. These more positivist aspects of the research design are a starting point for developing an understanding of the subjective empirical worlds of service users in the context of this study. We found greater explanatory power in the qualitative interview findings, both in what they revealed about what people liked and didn't like about their support services, and also in the symbols and meanings that were deployed. For example, it was clear that for the people running micro-enterprise services, to be 'a micro' referred to more than just their staff numbers: it was a shared identity that they had with other 'micros' across a local area. The term micro had normative power, a theme that is examined later in the book.

The critical-realist perspective felt particularly valuable because our literature review had revealed that many large n studies of organisational size and performance had inconclusive results. We felt an affinity with the insights of Skelcher that:

> the nearer a theoretical formulation approaches to an empirical reality, the less generalizable and hence the more trivial it becomes. The specifics of context ('the creation of the agency was enhanced by a major allocation of resources') and individual behaviour ('the new director was well-connected politically') squeeze out more generalizable and policy-relevant explanations of how public service performance is associated with the particular design of the organization's governance. (Skelcher, 2008, pp 39–40)

Skelcher's point is that 'governance and performance are understood as being enacted in a specific context, rather than being formal attributes of a system' (Skelcher, 2008, p 40), a conclusion with which we agree. Thus, although in the book we do offer generalisations to theory about organisational size and performance they are caveated in ways that we find more broadly necessary for social science research. The organisations in our study didn't sit still during the two years of our project: some expanded or shrank, some stopped trading, others grew so that they were no longer micros. We were interested in explaining this dynamic nature of size, rather than feeling that it rendered our independent variable too unstable to use it as the focus of enquiry.

Consistent with the reflexive approach to research that is demanded by critical realism, we acknowledge our role as researchers who are 'active reader[s]' and meaning-makers (Maynard-Moody and Musheno, 2003; Fischer, 2007; Yanow, 2007). As researchers we aim to 'tease out the argument implicitly embedded in the story' and to give a credible account of micro-enterprise, while recognising that 'different people construct different arguments out of the same narrative' (Fischer, 2003, p 181). We aimed to be alert to the ways in which policy actors interpret and shape meaning, but also to the ways in which we interpret those meanings. As Yanow puts it, '[W]e have a vision of a policy world that is made up of interpretations – and researchers themselves are also interpreters, making sense of policy documents along with oral policy language (e.g. speeches, interviews) and policy relevant acts' (Yanow, 2007, p 116).

Critical realism also commits us to research that is engaged with and seeks to influence social practices (Ackroyd and Karlsson, 2014, p 36). Each of us as authors comes with distinctive disciplinary identities (covering social policy, sociology, politics and public management), as well as our own normative framings on the appropriate balance between state and market provision in public services. Needham in particular has written critically on the consumerisation and privatisation of public services and the value of publicness (for example, Needham 2003, 2007). Micro-enterprises are arguably part of an outsourced (that is, non-public) care market. Yet they are also framed as being part of a community-oriented, asset-based alternative to large-scale privatisation. Much of the policy literature on micro-enterprises is highly normative, making explicit claims to be linked to new forms of community empowerment rather than simply a new delivery model (NAAPS, 2008; DH, 2010). During the early stages of the project, Community Catalysts, the national organisation that supports micro-enterprises, assisted us through brokering access to micro-enterprises in local sites that would not otherwise have been possible. We experienced at first hand the passion and commitment of those who see micro-enterprises as opening up ways for people to get support in ways that connect them to local communities.

In analysing the research findings and presenting them here as a way of informing care market development, we did not of course find that the politics of micro-enterprise could be easily fitted into a state good, market bad dichotomy. Micro-enterprises as an approach could be aligned to the New Left critique of state provision and the importance of local, community-based alternatives to state bureaucracies (Archer, 1989; Wainwright, 1994; Panitch and Leys, 2001). Again, though, this is not a wholly adequate account: some for-profit micro-enterprises have grown into small and medium-sized domiciliary care providers that to some extent look like any other market provider. The issues of micro-enterprise identity and growth are discussed in later chapters; we return to the politics of micro-enterprise in the final chapter.

Co-research

The project design encompassed a local asset-based approach to service users, working with cohorts of co-researchers in the three localities. A co-research approach was adopted in order to strengthen service user and carer perspectives throughout the study. This type of service user involvement is understood to have benefits for both the validity and relevance of research findings and for the individuals involved (Edwards and Alexander, 2011).

Twenty people were trained as co-researchers. They were recruited in the three localities and can be loosely grouped into two categories: people who use services, and people who are carers for people using services. These are recognised to be problematic labels, freezing identities into care giver and care receiver, whereas identities and relationships of dependence are much more fluid – an issue we return to later (Barnes et al, 2015).

Seventeen of the 20 co-researchers went on to lead research interviews, interpret and analyse data and disseminate findings (three left the project, due to alternative commitments or health issues). A particular asset the co-researchers brought to the study was their own local networks and service knowledge, which was often a tool for rapidly generating trust and accessing information in the interviews. The involvement of the co-researchers was evaluated at the end of the project by a team of researchers who had not been involved in the data-gathering process. The evaluation suggested benefits both for the individuals involved in co-research and for the research findings, as well as exploring a series of issues linked to the complexity of implementing co-research approaches – set out in more detail in Chapter Four.

Our pre-existing normative commitments to service user involvement were challenged while we were undertaking the research. As this was the first major project any of us had undertaken that aimed for substantive involvement by people with an experience of using care services, we had to address our own ambivalence about the way that this disrupted and challenged the usual flow of research (Flinders et al, 2015). Recruitment, training and involvement of older people, people with learning disabilities and carers led to ethical complexity, delays in starting the fieldwork and a myriad of unexpected issues during the interviews themselves (which were undertaken jointly by the co-researcher and academic researcher). The people we were interviewing, for example, didn't always welcome the presence of someone from their 'own community', when they had agreed to take part in a university research project and expected to be interviewed by someone who 'looked like' a researcher. These points are not meant in any way to critique the contribution of the co-researchers – rather, they affirm our own messy and unfinished process of learning to be co-productive researchers.

Outline of the book

Following this introductory chapter, Chapters Two and Three situate the research in the policy context and academic literature to establish the importance of taking size seriously within public services. Five themed literature reviews were undertaken at the start of the research in order to align how the research team understood the policy context, to develop the research hypotheses and to inform the research design. Topics covered in these reviews were: the relationship between organisational size and performance; the policy context and outcomes associated with social care services; the role of micro-enterprises and the third sector in public service provision; the provision available for seldom-heard groups in the community; and participatory approaches to research. Literature for the reviews was drawn from a combination of search techniques including systematic database searching and snowball sampling. We took a narrative approach to the review, informed by Greenhalgh and Peacock's (2005) model of searching for complex evidence, including non-systematically derived sources, which they describe as serendipitous.

Chapter Two examines the issue of why size is a relevant frame to use in relation to performance and innovation in public services, outlining key findings from the existing literature. In recognition of the inconclusive nature of efforts to find relationships between size and performance or size and innovation, three further aspects of size are discussed. First, size is recognised to be a dynamic variable that is constantly shifting, and measurable in a range of different ways that impede comparative analysis. Second, size is recognised to have a symbolic and performative aspect, which needs to be part of an understanding of the way that it behaves as a research variable. Third is the distinctive context of care. We set out recent reforms to social care services in the era since the care management reforms of the early 1990s. This covers the move to large-scale outsourcing of care services as well as the more recent shift to personalisation and cost cutting as the driving rationales for service delivery.

Chapter Three focuses on enterprise and care, considering the contribution that new delivery models such as social enterprises make within public services more broadly and care in particular. The chapter also considers the ambiguity of the social-enterprise label and its capacity to be claimed by a range of governance types, including the for-profit as well as the not-for-profit. The chapter then draws together the evidence on micro-enterprises into four research hypotheses that are tested in later chapters of the book.

Chapters Four and Five are concerned with research methods; however, we present these not as a throat-clearing exercise before the 'real findings' start in Chapter Six, but as ways to explicate two substantive aspects of the work. Chapter Four focuses on involving people using and working in care services as co-researchers, framing each stage of the research process as one in which we had to depart from our planned approach and think about doing research differently. We locate it in the context of existing research on the increasingly significant issue of co-production of research with people who may be considered 'beneficiaries' of the research, that is, people with an experience of using services and family carers. Co-produced research is often presented as an unalloyed good, given its commitment to sharing power with potentially marginalised groups whose expertise can improve the research and give it more legitimacy within affected communities. However, more critical accounts of co-produced research are also emerging (for example, Flinders et al's (2015) description of its potential to be a 'pollution' of academic research) that at the very least require a more considered defence of its importance.

Chapter Five is a discussion of what it means to be a micro-enterprise, outlining the approach taken to sampling and accessing the case study organisations, the different governance types included and the meanings that interviewees attached to different types and sizes of organisation. It affirms that the question of what it means to be micro was partly answered by the research team in the approach that we took to sampling (FTE staff numbers), but is also located within the organisational identities expressed by people from different sizes and types of provider.

Chapters Six, Seven and Eight can more straightforwardly be identified as research-findings chapters, in which we draw on primary data generated from the research to explain what it tells us in relation to the hypotheses about micro care providers (the extent to which micro-enterprises deliver more valued outcomes, are more cost-effective, more personalised and more innovative than larger providers). Chapter Six examines issues relating to the outcomes of care, bringing in the formal outcomes data from ASCOT. We also discuss here the pricing data from the organisations in our study, drawing conclusions about value for money by comparing price and outcome data. We contextualise these findings in broader debates about how care is financed, and the fit between micro-enterprises and individualised purchasing by personal budget holders and people who fund their own care.

An outcomes orientation can be described as taking a 'black box' approach that does not explain how outcomes are achieved (Behn, 2003). Chapters Seven and Eight look inside this black box at the process of care, in order to explain how far services are personalised and innovative. Chapter Seven discusses the enactment of personalisation, highlighting the ways in which very small organisations seem to be able to adapt more flexibly to people's desire for sustained and trusting relationships in a care context. In Chapter Eight, we draw out three types of innovation – *what* innovation, *how* innovation and *who* innovation – and argue that micro-enterprises are best at offering *how* and *who* innovation. New types of service (the *what* innovations) were less evident in our findings, and micro-enterprises were no more likely to offer these than the larger providers in our sample.

Chapter Nine considers a range of explanations as to why micro-enterprises perform well on aspects of all of the four measures that we used (valued, cost-effective, personalised and innovative). It focuses on the organisational structure of micro-enterprises, suggesting that their size allows these organisations to foster staff autonomy and high levels of adaptability to what is wanted by the people they support. It also examines issues of organisational ethos and identity, suggesting that many of these organisations set themselves up explicitly to distinguish themselves from large providers, and that this is the driver for much of the personalised support and innovative practice that we saw. However, there are also vulnerabilities here for these organisations that can lack financial security, raising question marks about their long-term sustainability. Chapter Ten considers these issues, exploring micro-enterprise funding models, which rely heavily on individualised purchasing by people rather than on local government contracts. The chapter also considers how these organisations interact with the local authority and the regulator. It argues that micro-enterprises retain a reliance on formal institutions within the care system – local authorities, the CQC – that can limit their scope to 'break the mould' when it comes to care and support.

Chapter Eleven, the concluding chapter, considers the implications of the findings for the future of English social care services and for the broader health and welfare system. It suggests that local care economies are complex adaptive systems in which niche organisations like micro-enterprises can thrive but in which local authorities have weak coordinating tools to support micro-enterprise development. The employment of designated micro-enterprise coordinators within local authorities can enhance support for micro-enterprises, but even in localities with coordinators the micro-enterprises remain fragile. We also consider whether the benefits of 'smallness' can be achieved through other means than micro-enterprises, discussing what can be learned from examples of large organisations that have found ways to nest smaller units within them. These discussions suggest opportunities for further research, particularly longitudinal and internationally comparative research, that stretch the impact of our findings beyond the time-scale and geographical reach of our current study.

The book finishes by returning to the politics of micro-enterprise. Care and enterprise are not necessarily practices and attitudes that are easily aligned, and we do not seek to endorse an approach in which those giving and receiving care have to reinvent themselves as entrepreneurs. However, the experience of doing the research has highlighted the poor quality of some large-scale provision – particularly in home care – and the benefits that very small-scale organisations, working within their own local communities, can bring.

TWO

Why study size?

To understand the extent to which micro-enterprises in the care sector perform better than larger care providers requires a sensitivity to issues relating to size and to the growth of enterprise within public services. The first of these issues is the focus of this chapter; the second is discussed in Chapter Three. This chapter uses size as a lens through which to examine performance and innovation within public services. Shifting fashions in the optimal size of public organisations have been central to the history of public administration. Weber's (1997) theory of bureaucracy prized the economies of scale and coordination offered by large organisations. New Public Management-type reforms sought to disaggregate large bureaucracies into smaller, self-managed units, efficiently focused on a specific task (Hood, 1991). Subsequent approaches, sometimes captured under the heading of 'new public governance' (Osborne, 2010), have emphasised joining back up through partnerships, networks and collaboration, if not formal mergers (Rhodes, 1997; Kooiman, 2003).

Through presenting existing research on organisational size, performance and innovation, the chapter draws attention to a paradox: research studies repeatedly affirm that it is difficult to establish a relationship between organisational size and performance or between size and innovation. However policy makers continue to play with size, in the anticipation that it will make organisations perform better or be more innovative. The chapter goes on to examine why size continues to matter, highlighting the limitations of approaches to size that focus on linear relationships between stable variables. Size is constantly shifting and subject to a range of different definitions. Of course, most terms within social science are unstable, but other organisational features – governance arrangements, for example – are better defined, legally bounded and likely to be more stable than organisational size. We must be alert to the symbolic and performative elements of size, which help to explain why size continues to play an important role in public service redesign. Having discussed these aspects, the chapter goes on to examine the role that size plays in different service sectors, highlighting the distinctiveness of the context of care.

Organisational size and performance

The extent to which small organisations perform better than larger ones has been a core question for economic theory and business studies, as well as for public management. Commentators have noted the tendency for cycling between assumptions that large organisations deliver better outcomes (through economies of scale and integrated communication) and that small organisations are better, since they can be more autonomous and specialised (Boyne, 2003a; Pollitt, 2003; Talbot and Johnson, 2006). On the side of small organisations sit classic texts such as Schumacher's *Small is Beautiful*, with its critique of growth as inherently desirable, or more recently Boyle's (2011) *The Human Element*, which argues that small organisations outperform large ones on productivity, cost and innovation. Harrison's *Lean and Mean* (1997) exemplifies the counter-argument, citing the greater adaptability and durability of large companies. Economic theory, as Boyne summarises, 'suggests that the benefits of organizational growth will eventually be offset by costs such as managerial overheads and bureaucratic rigidity' (Boyne, 2003a, pp 382–3). Within the business literature, there has been some confirmation of this inverted U-shape pattern, with medium-sized organisations being found in some studies to offer the optimum combination of flexibility and resilience (for example, Haveman, 2003).

In entering this debate, it helps to narrow the focus to the public management literature, given the distinctive political and financial context in which public service organisations operate. The various definitions of performance that proliferate in the public management literature are distilled by Boyne (2002, 2003a) into the following six measures of performance for public service organisations:

- quantity of outputs (such as number of operations performed in a hospital)
- quality of outputs (such as speed and reliability of service)
- efficiency (ratio of outputs to financial inputs)
- value for money (cost per unit of outcome)
- outcomes (such as percentage of patients treated successfully)
- consumer satisfaction (which may be a proxy for other measures).

Boyne notes that different stakeholders will attach different weight to the six measures and that the weight they attach to each one is likely to vary and to shift over time (Boyne, 2003a, p 368). Some of them are 'objective' measures, in that they can be measured against standard benchmarks: quantity of outputs and efficiency fall into this category. Others have a 'subjective' aspect to them, in that they involve stakeholder perception (Andrews et al, 2012). These include outcomes and consumer satisfaction. Objective and subjective measures can be combined to give a picture of organisational performance, although they may not always report the same results (Andrews et al, 2012). Andrews et al see objective and subjective measures of performance as 'different pieces of the performance jigsaw. They are rarely measures of precisely the same elements of performance, so it is unsurprising that they are not closely correlated' (Andrews et al, 2012, p 32).

Boyne identifies five theories about what drives improved performance across the six measures: resources, regulation, market structure, management and organisation (which includes organisational size). Systematically reviewing 65 quantitative studies in academic journals of the impact of one of more of these factors on service improvement, he finds that greater resources and better management have a positive influence on performance, whereas for the other theories the evidence is 'thin or contradictory' (Boyne, 2003a). Organisational size – defined variously in the studies as the general population in a locality, staff, capacity and number of service users – is not found to be a significant determinant of performance. Summarising the results of 18 studies that have tested for a linear relationship between organisational size and performance, Boyne concludes:

> The results offer little comfort to the advocates of large or small organizations: around two-thirds of the size coefficients are insignificant ... Furthermore the impact of size does not appear to be linked systematically to type of service (e.g. schools) or specific dimensions of performance (e.g. output quantity or outcomes). (Boyne, 2003a, pp 382–3)

Boyne's conclusion that there is no linear relationship between size and performance is consistent with other reviews. For example, Peckham et al's review of the literature on decentralisation within health services found that 'size is only one of a number of factors that shape performance ... The idea that there is an optimal size is a fantasy; multiple functions mean organisations need to compromise between different optimal sizes for each function' (Peckham et al, 2005). As Sheaff et al put it, reporting on a systematic review of organisational size in healthcare: 'Different organisational sizes appear optimal for different processes. There is no evidence suggesting a single "best size" for each kind of organisation' (Sheaff et al, 2004, p 97).

Boyne also reviews the studies of non-linear relationships between size and organisational performance and finds that these have produced a greater percentage of significant results than studies that have examined only linear size effects. However, 'the pattern in the evidence is complex: almost as many tests indicate that performance at first falls with size and then eventually rises as indicate the reverse ... Thus whether reformers are better advised to break up large public agencies or amalgamate small ones remains unclear' (Boyne, 2003a, p 385). These studies highlight the complexity of the relationship between size and performance and the difficulties of drawing generalisable conclusions.

Size and innovation

The propensity to innovate is another management feature that may be deployed differently in organisations of different sizes. Walker (2008) defines innovation as 'a process through which new ideas, objects and practices are created, developed or reinvented, and are new for the unit of adoption' (cited in Williams, 2010). One of the original and most comprehensive conceptualisations of innovation was by Schumpeter (1934), who defined innovation in five ways: the introduction of new goods, new methods of production, the opening of new markets, the conquest of new sources of supply or the reorganisation of an industry. This and subsequent definitions of innovation focus their attention on the process of creation, development and implementation of new ideas (Camison Zornoza et al, 2004; Walker, 2014). Social innovations have also been differentiated from business innovations; while business innovations are normally driven by profit maximisation and are diffused through profit-driven organisations, social innovations tend to occur in response to worsening social problems, when systems are not working and when there are gaps in existing provision by governments (or the private sector) (Mulgan, 2007).

There have been numerous attempts to relate innovation to organisation size; however, this relationship remains open to debate, making it difficult to theorise whether micro-enterprises will be more innovative than larger care services. On one side of the debate, much of the literature indicates a positive relationship between size and innovation (Camison Zornoza et al, 2004; Greenhalgh et al, 2004), meaning that larger organisations are more likely to display innovation than are smaller organisations. This is because larger organisations have more resources, including more professional, skilled workers, access to complex facilities and higher technical knowledge, enabling them to adopt a higher number of innovations (Damanpour and Evan, 1984; Camison Zornoza et al, 2004; Damanpour et al, 2009). Large organisations are also able to take on greater risks and better able to bear the losses brought about when innovations are not successful (Damanpour, 1992; Hitt et al, 1997; Camison Zornoza et al, 2004). Daft and Becker (1978) argue that larger organisations provide the support, leadership and coordination required for innovations to succeed. This is supported in a systematic review by Greenhalgh et al (2004, p 212):

> one of the most commonly observed findings about organisational innovation is the positive correlation with large size ... Rather than size per se, explanations include that larger size increases the likelihood that other predictors of innovation will be present, including the availability of financial and human resources (organisational slack) and differentiation or specialisation.

Other research has found a negative relationship between size and innovation. From this perspective, the inherent advantage of small organisations is their flexibility, allowing them to adapt, as well as accept and implement changes more readily (Damanpour, 1996). The formal and bureaucratic structures of large organisations can make them resistant to change and innovation (Van de Venn and Rogers, 1988; Scherer and Ross 1990). Large public organisations have been argued to be particularly resistant to consumer-responsive innovation, being driven by the interests of bureaucrats rather than users (Downs, 1967; Niskanen, 1971).

Alternatively, a third body of research indicates no relationship between size and innovation, pointing to other factors as better indicators of propensity to innovate (Aiken et al, 1980; Camison Zornoza et al, 2004). These inconsistencies in the research findings may in part be explained by methodological differences in how innovation and size are defined and measured (for example, by number of employees, financial resources/outputs) (Damanpour, 1992). Walker (2014, p 25) argues that these conflicting theoretical viewpoints indicate a possible non-linear relationship between innovation and size, 'with both smaller and larger organisations offering optimal structural conditions for innovation'. Indeed it may be that both large and small organisations can mimic the advantages of the other to foster innovation. Quinn (1985) suggests that large organisations can establish subunits that 'behave like small entrepreneurial ventures (that is, work semi–autonomously, thereby being freed of bureaucratic constraints) while at the same time enjoying the benefits (buffering of cash flow, for example) offered by a larger company' (cited in Greenhalgh et al, 2004, p 212). Conversely, research on 'creative clusters' has suggested that small organisations can co-locate with other similar bodies to reduce isolation and create synergies that catalyse innovation (Chapain et al, 2010).

Bringing size back in

Despite the inconclusive evidence base set out above relating to the impact of size on performance or innovation, the resizing of public service delivery organisations has been an almost constant focus for policy makers' energies. As suggested earlier, it is possible to identify cycling over time between preferences for large and small organisations (Boyne, 1996; Pollitt, 2008). Although the cycles have been evident in a large number of developed states, the focus and periodisation has been somewhat different. Within the UK, where the influence of Weber was less pronounced than elsewhere, Fabian principles of bureaucratic efficiency underpinned the development of large government welfare departments in the 20th century (Webb and Webb, 1920; Clarke et al, 1987). As Boyne puts it:

> Large units were expected to provide services more efficiently because the employment of specialist staff and equipment would be more feasible at higher levels of output. Also, bigger organizations would find it easier to distribute services across large client groups and thereby ensure reliability and equity of provision. (Boyne, 1996, p 811)

By the 1970s these assumptions were coming under attack from 'New Right' politicians who had discovered public choice theory (for example, Joseph, 1975). The New Public Management-type (NPM) approaches that followed were based on the hypothesis 'that there is a negative relationship between scale and performance' (Boyne, 1996). A presumption that efficiency was enhanced through specialisation led to the creation by government of arm's-length agencies and the privatisation of welfare services to make them more results focused and responsive to their publics (Hood, 1991).

The perceived fragmentation caused by these changes ensured that by the 1990s there were calls from government and academics for 'joining back up' (Cabinet Office, 1999; Rhodes, 1997; Rainey and Steinbauer, 1999). While this did not prompt a return to large government bureaucracies, it encouraged organisations to work more collaboratively, in loose partnerships and networks, rather than operating as small, isolated units. The autonomy of the separate agencies fostered in the earlier period was also quashed by increasingly prescriptive regulation regimes, demanding standardised practices from local government and providers (Gray and Jenkins, 2011).

A more recent vogue for personalised approaches within welfare services has emerged in the 21st century. It has not replaced either the fragmented patchwork of collaborating agencies and providers, or the standardised regulatory context, but awkwardly coexists with both. Service providers seem to be expected to be able to deliver 'standards not standardisation'. The Coalition government (2010–15) and the Conservative government from 2015 have sent ambivalent signals about what size of service provider is preferred. The 'Big Society' rhetoric seemed to favour small community social enterprises, while procurement and commissioning practices have rewarded larger organisations (McCabe and Phillimore, 2012), a theme discussed further in the next chapter.

These cyclical patterns highlight the ongoing fascination that policy makers have with playing with scale as a way to improve performance. As Postma puts it, 'policy makers, executives and other actors have high expectations of the relation between (changes in) scale and positive outcomes, like quality and efficiency of care' (Postma, 2015, p 12). They believe in and strive for the 'optimal scale' (Postma, 2015, p 15). Such an observation highlights the extent to which size and scale operate as discursive framings as well as organisational characteristics, and can be understood through social–constructionist accounts of organisational performance as well as testable variables in empirical studies. In discursive or interpretive accounts of performance, attention is paid to organisational image and legitimacy rather than formal input or output measures. Writing about governance, Skelcher suggests: 'what is important is not performance per se, but the ability of different interests to attribute or explain that performance in terms of the form of public governance preferred by each' (Skelcher, 2008, p 38). Noting the tendency of quantitative studies of performance to produce inconclusive results and/or organisation-specific findings from which it is very difficult to generalise, he calls for a 'new entry point', drawing on interpretivist approaches, that recognises that 'discourses validate particular forms of governance in terms of their performance, and thus guide the practices of actors' (Skelcher, 2008, p 40). Focusing on scale, Postma similarly suggests that scale is a social construction, 'an outcome of the interplay between the multiple interests, values and perceptions of the people that are involved and broader social and political processes' (Postma, 2015, p 19).

Pursuing discursive understandings of size and performance requires a rethinking not only of performance but also of organisations as fixed and stable entities. Sheaff's systematic review of devolution of health services, cited above, begins with a definition of an organisation as 'a concrete, observable association of persons engaged in collective activities and pursuing common objectives' (Sheaff et al, 2004). However, this perspective has been challenged by two different literatures. The first, a social-constructivist account, suggests that organisations are most appropriately seen as bundles of processes in perpetual motion, rather than as bounded entities (for example, Tsoukas and Chia (2002)). Organisations come into being in the ways that they are narrated (Czarniawska, 1997). Selecting and studying the unit of analysis brings one version of the organisation to the fore while others fall away.

Second, within the mainstream management literature the notion of a firm as a singular, integrated structure has been challenged by the emergence of 'modular organisations' in which:

> the locus of production is no longer within the boundaries of a single firm, but occurs instead at the nexus of relationships between a variety of parties that contribute to the production function ... The loosely coupled organizational forms allow organizational components to be flexibly recombined into a variety of configurations. (Schilling and Steensma, 2001, p 1149)

Both these literatures highlight that the way that an organisation is summoned and narrated by policy makers and academics requires choices (the ways that we engaged with those choices in our sampling of micro-enterprises is discussed in Chapter Five). In exploring the relationship between size and desirable traits such as high performance and innovation, it highlights that policy actors have choices in the ways in which they describe and measure organisations, and that these will shape the extent to which particular organisational forms are viewed as effective. As Andrews et al put it: 'An organisation is perceived as legitimate by powerful stakeholders if its internal arrangements are consistent with prevailing norms (in other words, it is managed in a way that is "modern" or "fashionable")' (Andrews et al, 2012). For example, the political support for social enterprise as an organisational form in the last ten years has led, argue Teasdale et al (2013), to a vast inflation in the numbers of such enterprises recorded in official statistics: 'as the language of social enterprise ... has infiltrated popular discourse, more individuals are aware of the social desirability or normative legitimacy attached to self-identifying with this definition. Whether this growth reflects any real change in organisational behaviour is far from clear' (Teasdale et al, 2013, p 128).

There is an epistemological point here about the ways in which the relationship between organisational characteristics and performance is socially constructed. There is also, in Andrews et al's use of the term 'fashionable' a reminder that organisations that are viewed as effective have to strike a balance: fashion is about fitting in with prevailing norms (isomorphism – Powell and DiMaggio, 2012), but also about emphasising divergence from other social groups (Veblen, 1970). Macmillan's work on distinction in the third sector highlights that categories of organisation (the third sector, for example) have to make a claim to distinctiveness. Applying the work of Bourdieu to the third sector, Macmillan notes that 'the strategic purpose of claims to distinctiveness, has been overlooked in recent debates on the sector' (2013, p 40). He explains:

> Organisations are ultimately placed in a competitive relationship with each other for various forms of capital, even though much of this rivalry is disguised, implied or latent. In this context claims for uniqueness or distinctiveness become *strategies of distinction*, designed to create or preserve room for individual third sector organisations (against other organisations), groups of like-minded third sector organisations (against other groups), and the third sector as a whole (against other sectors). (Macmillan, 2013, p 42, emphasis in original)

For organisations to be viewed as performing well, therefore, it may be necessary to convince stakeholders of both their fit and their distinctiveness.

Such approaches take us a long way away from the internal variables of performance that were covered in Boyne's (2003a) meta-review, challenging the notion of stable and measurable aspects of organisational characteristics and performance. Boyne himself suggests that what he calls contingent approaches should be part of the toolkit, but they should not be a replacement for measuring tangible elements of service standards (speed, quality, reliability). He sets out a combination of goal-related measurement and discursive approaches as follows: 'a working definition of improvement must incorporate both the substance of organizational achievements, and the inherently political nature of judgements on success or failure' (Boyne, 2003b). Similarly Talbot (2010) identifies the advantages of combining formal performance measures with symbolic aspects when studying organisational performance.

The relationship between organisational size and dependent variables such as performance and innovation can then be examined through a combined approach: by looking at the interplay of variables through empirical measurement, and through examining the normative framings surfaced by more interpretive approaches. Distilling the discussion above for its implications for micro-enterprises, then, there is an imperative to establish effectiveness on a number of criteria: the formal measures of performance which remain part of building a case for legitimacy with commissioners and potential clients; an ability to fit with the prevailing norms in relation to organisational size; and an ability to establish a distinctive offer. These different aspects of effectiveness are returned to in later chapters. The section below examines the relationship between organisational size, performance and innovation in a care setting.

What is the right size for care?

It is necessary to consider how such debates play out within particular service contexts, recognising that optimal scales for schools (the focus for many of the quantitative studies in Boyne's (2003a) meta-review of size and performance) may have limited read across for health and social care services. Sector-specific research can draw attention to the ways in which norms of convergence and distinction are constructed in relation to particular types of service. Postma's work on Dutch healthcare provides a good example of shifting norms in relation to organisational size. Analysing newspaper reporting of scale in Dutch healthcare over a quarter-century, he found that:

> Over time and throughout the different discourses, actors increasingly favour small organizational scale and oppose large organizational scale. More and more, large-scale was associated with distance, inefficiency, bureaucracy and overpaid management. On the other hand, small-scale was associated with values like proximity, affordability,

recognition, professional freedom and humanity. Exceptions
were executives of healthcare organizations, who over
time favour large organizational scale. They argued that
large-scale care is needed to achieve a good market
position, provide efficient and integrated care and stimulate
professional development. (Postma, 2015, p 98)

Although equivalent research is not available for the UK, the divergent
perspectives that Postma identified do resonate, in that health and
social care discourses on preferred scales are proceeding in different
directions. Since 2007, for example, the focus from policy leaders
in social care has been to emphasise the benefits of personalised
care, tailored to the individual and delivered where possible by small
community organisations (for example, Putting People First, 2007).
Within health, there has been more optimism about the efficiency and
safety of large organisations, such as the creation of so-called 'super-
practices' for general practitioners and the concentration of surgical
specialties in larger hospital settings (National Audit Office, 2010; Smith
et al, 2013). This, though, has been allied with a different message
for people assessed as having both health and social care needs over
the longer term. Integrated approaches for the treatment of people
with long-term conditions have invoked the importance of 'whole
person' approaches that are more focused on small-scale, individualised
interventions (Bickerstaffe, 2013; NHS, 2014).

A key driver of the focus on smaller-scale interventions in social
care has been the personalisation agenda. Driven by a goal to
promote independence and choice in adult social care (DH, 2005),
the introduction of 'personalisation' has attempted to return the
control of purchasing care services to the service user. Emerging from
the *Putting People First* concordat of 2007 (although with a longer
genealogy in campaigns for independent living and direct payments),
the personalisation reform agenda has emphasised the need to tailor
services to the individual (Needham, 2011). The agenda has four
strands through which to realise person-centred social care: offering
choice and control; investing in prevention; building social capital;
enhancing access to universal services (Putting People First, 2007). Of
these, it is the development of personal budgets (part of the choice-
and-control strand) that has been the most high-profile aspect (Glasby
and Littlechild, 2016).

Personal budgets can be taken in the form of 'direct payments',
which are a cash sum provided to the disabled person in lieu of
services provided (Glasby and Littlechild, 2016), making the service

user both the purchaser and consumer of care. Alternatively, personal budgets can be managed by the local authority, allowing the personal-budget holder to choose how some or all of it is spent but leaving the council to commission services. The ambition to make people 'individual commissioners' and to reduce the number of large contracts commissioned by the local authority has gained new impetus following the Care Act 2014.

Much of the rationale for the personalisation message comes from a sense that social care is for intensely personal matters (washing, dressing, deciding how to spend the day), where care providers need to be able to operate on an interpersonal and responsive level. The social-innovation network In Control, which has worked with local authorities to promote and support the take-up of personal budgets, emphasises, 'it's about giving people real power and control over their lives' (In Control, no date a).

Personalisation, then, can be seen as requiring organisations that can work on a 'human scale', which Postma (2015, p 99) defines in the following way:

> The human scale discourse entails such words as 'home', 'neighbourhood', 'human', 'care' and 'community'. The discourse demarcates the space that patients, clients and citizens inhabit as the scale that is most relevant ... 'lived experiences' in everyday lives of patients, are central in this discourse. (Postma, 2015, pp 99–100)

The foregrounding of home and neighbourhood is reinforced by growing trends to keep people in their own homes for longer, rather than moving into residential care (House of Lords, 2013). Enthusiasm for large-scale residential provision within the care sector has been weakened by the exposure of abuse within institutions, which has been a recurrent theme since the Ely hospital scandal of the late 1960s. Such cases have led disability campaigners such as Duffy to passionately denounce institutionalisation (Duffy, 2014). Outside of specific cases of abuse, there has been a widespread rejection of the segregated model offered by large institutions, in favour of small group homes and more independent approaches (Goffman, 1968; Cambridge et al, 1994; Holman, 1996).

Personalisation is premised on a range of services existing in the market for people with personal budgets to choose from, thereby bridging the gap between what people want and what is supplied. One way in which the supply of social care services has been expanded and diversified is through micro-enterprises that claim to provide choice and individualised solutions at a small scale (NAAPS, 2008). The importance of micro-enterprise in delivering choice for people with personal budgets has been argued for some time and was highlighted in the White Paper *Caring for our future: Reforming care and support* (DH, 2012). The White Paper emphasised the way in which small, user-led organisations, for example, could support the diversification of the social care market. While large block contracts previously favoured large providers and economies of scale, personalisation may remove the monopolistic tendencies of this system. Smaller social care providers, including micro-enterprises that struggle to compete for large contracts, could benefit from an increase in the number of individual purchasers (Baxter et al, 2011). Personalisation should makes it easier for new, smaller providers to enter the market because, rather than looking to secure large contracts (which require significant inputs of money and skills), providers can build capacity one client at a time (Baxter et al, 2011). Personalisation may also bring opportunities for existing providers to diversify their activities in line with the needs of older and disabled people, who may want something more varied than traditional personal care. This provides opportunities to enter new service areas, such as the delivery of social activities or help with shopping.

The Care Act gave local authorities market-shaping duties to stimulate this small-scale local provision, as it came to be seen that personal budgets themselves would not stimulate a market to emerge. Social care is often arranged at a time of crisis, such as upon leaving hospital, and people in such a vulnerable situation may not be in a position to make a decision about how a personal budget should be spent (Lloyd, 2010). Subsequently, while 76% of eligible people now hold a personal budget to pay for care, over two-thirds of these are managed personal budgets (held by the local authority) rather than direct payments to the service user (Samuel, 2013). Take-up by older people is especially low (Age UK, 2013). It has been argued that frail older people may struggle to exercise the control and choice central to the policy and instead prefer a third party to arrange their care package (Brindle, 2008; Glendinning et al, 2008). In this context, local authorities may default to using large-scale providers with whom they have framework contracts, rather than helping people to access small-scale support.

Conclusion

It can be seen, then, that the interplay between organisational size and performance or innovation has been the focus of many studies, with inconclusive results. Perceived links between size and performance have been the driver of much government reform, given the preference of NPM-inspired reformers for small, discrete service-provider units over large, multi-purpose bureaucracies. Size of organisation continues to be a variable that governments emphasise when considering how to optimise service performance. Although the high-water mark of NPM has now passed, faith that changing the size of providers will improve performance remains high. Size therefore cannot be written off as a research focus, given its symbolic allure and the ways in which differently sized organisations can make a claim to fit or distinctiveness as a way of making space for themselves within the terrain of public services.

The chapter has also discussed social care as a sector with distinctive features that give size a particular resonance. The 'human scale' of very small services may be particularly apt for a setting in which interpersonal relationships are a key aspect of what constitutes good quality. In particular, the personalisation reforms in social care services that have followed the longer-term project of outsourcing care from the public sector have created an imperative in which the person rather than the organisation should become the relevant unit of analysis. However, the slow progress on implementation of more individualised commissioning has limited the development of small-scale care provision to date.

The next chapter considers the context of enterprise within public services, and focuses more specifically on enterprise-based approaches to the delivery of care services. Four hypotheses about the benefits of micro-enterprises are considered.

THREE

Enterprise and care

Since the 1990s there have been far-reaching reforms to public services in England, resulting in less direct state provision of public service and an increased marketisation of the public sector through the outsourcing of services to a range of competing providers (McKay et al, 2011; Hazenberg and Hall, 2014). This commitment to a diversity of welfare provision has fostered a 'mixed economy of welfare', increasing the role of the third and private sectors as providers of public services (Powell, 2007).

This chapter considers changes to social care since the 1990s, which have culminated in the bulk of care being delivered outside of the statutory sector, a development that more recently has been overlaid by a commitment to personalised care services. The chapter also looks more broadly at the encouragement of social enterprise by government, particularly since 2010 when the Conservative party took power, first in coalition and then as a single-party majority government. The chapter then goes on to consider micro-enterprises in particular, setting out their key features. It considers the claims that are made about such enterprises in a care context and uses these as the basis of four research hypotheses.

Marketising social care

English social care took its current form from the National Assistance Act 1948, although it has longer antecedents in the workhouse culture of the Victorian Poor Law (Birch, 1974). Prior to the 1970s, responsibility for personal social services was dispersed between different local government branches and the NHS (Kirkpatrick, 2006). Following recommendations from the 1968 Seebohm Report, the early 1970s saw a consolidation of the system and the formation of unified social services departments within local government. Local authorities took responsibility for planning and delivering services, with a limited role being played by independent organisations.

As part of broader public management changes under the Thatcher governments, the NHS and Community Care Act 1990 established a mixed economy framework for service provision within adult social care (Baxter et al, 2011). Local authorities were urged to move away from providing their social care services 'in-house' and instead to purchase provision from private and voluntary sector providers on behalf of service users. This was justified by the Conservative government at the time, as well as subsequent New Labour governments, on the grounds that the development of a social care market subject to competition would stimulate diversity within social care provision, ensuring more choice for users, while also providing greater cost-effectiveness (Kirkpatrick, 2006). The 1990s saw a transition of care provision from the state to the independent sector, such that by 1999 local authorities were buying more care from the independent sector than they provided themselves (Scourfield, 2006). By 2012, the independent sector accounted for almost three-quarters (72%) of all social care provision (Skills for Care, 2013).

During the 1990s, local authority contracts for social care tended to be in the form of short-term 'spot' contracts of a specified set of services for an individual. While spot purchasing provided flexibility in commissioning, it was criticised for creating financial uncertainty among providers, as contracted organisations were unable to plan ahead and recruit staff for the long term (Scourfield, 2006). This in turn was felt to contribute to low pay and inadequate staff training within the independent social care sector (Kirkpatrick, 2006). In the late 1990s local authorities began to develop more collaborative relationships with independent sector providers. This led to approved lists of favoured providers and a move to longer-term 'block' contracts (Kirkpatrick, 2006). Local authorities could pre-buy a determined number of hours of care at a discounted cost, using economies-of-scale principles. While this offered greater security to providers who could employ staff on a longer-term basis, block contracts have also been criticised for creating local monopolies of large providers, limiting the diversity of social care services and, ultimately, choice for service users (Baxter et al, 2011). Such practices also limit the ability of small care services to enter the market and compete for contracts.

More recent social care reform emerged from the Care Act 2014, which sets out new duties for local authorities and new rights for social care users and family carers. The Act states that local authorities are required to develop a diverse social care market that delivers a wide range of high-quality care and support services. Local authorities are also required to encourage a range of providers and services from the private sector and the voluntary and community sector, including user-led organisations, social enterprises, mutuals and small businesses (DH, 2014). It seems likely that, as a result of this legal duty and the broader context of personalisation that was discussed in the previous chapter, local authorities will look to broaden out from a small number of block-commissioned providers and encourage smaller enterprises to enter the care sector.

Social enterprise

Social enterprises have no fixed definition or legal form, and the name has been appropriated by a range of organisational types as highlighted in the previous chapter (Teasdale, 2011). However, they have been broadly defined as 'business[es] with primarily social objectives whose surpluses are principally reinvested for that purpose in the business or in the community, rather than being driven by the need to maximise profit for shareholders and owners' (DTI, 2002). There is no pre-ordained governance model for a social enterprise and they take many forms, including sole traders, partnerships, limited companies with charitable status, industrial and provident societies, co-operatives and mutuals. In an attempt to rectify this lack of clarity, the Community Interest Company (CIC) was introduced in 2004, offering a specific legal organisational form for social enterprises, although social enterprises are not required to become CICs.

Whereas the Thatcher and Major governments (1979–97) assumed a fairly binary distinction between the for-profit and not-for-profit sectors, under New Labour (1997–2010) the notion of social enterprise increasingly came to be seen as offering a 'third way' in public service outsourcing, combining market principles of business with the social values of the third sector (Teasdale, 2011). Social enterprise later came to be particularly associated with David Cameron's attempt to articulate a new kind of Conservatism after he became party leader in 2005. The Conservatives in the run-up to the 2010 election developed a flagship 'Big Society' agenda, which for a while became the animating principle of the Conservative–Liberal Democrat coalition that took power. The stated aim of the Big Society agenda was 'to create a climate that empowers local people and communities, building a big society that will take power away from politicians and give it to people' (Cabinet Office, 2010a, 2010b). Principles included community empowerment, decentralised services, increased volunteerism and greater support for the third sector (Alcock, 2010; Cabinet Office, 2010b; DH, 2010; Needham, 2011; Rees and Mullins, 2016).

The Big Society rhetoric did not last long (Jeffares, 2014) and was largely abandoned by the time of the 2015 general election. However, a lasting legacy that is relevant for our research was the support it gave to social enterprise models of public service delivery. In 2010, the Coalition government's programme for government stated:

> [We will] support the creation and expansion of mutuals, co-operatives, charities and social enterprises, and enable these groups to have a much greater involvement in the running of public services. (HM Government, 2010)

Policies to increase the supply of community and third sector services included the Localism Act 2011, which provided opportunities for community groups to take over and run their local services. Under this Act, the 'Community Right to Challenge' gave voluntary or community bodies, charities, parish councils or local authority staff the right to express an interest in running local authority services (Department for Communities and Local Government, 2012).

Social enterprises now provide many public services that are financed through government contracts. The key benefits claimed for social enterprise include greater staff control and increased user participation, which results in services that are more innovative and responsive (Hazenberg and Hall, 2014). Social enterprises tie in with the broader co-production agenda, as they are seen as having a 'commitment to deliver high quality services, a desire to empower their staff and place the communities and people they serve at their core' (DH, 2008a, p 5).

An area of public service in which social enterprise plays a particularly significant role is health and social care. The NHS Next Stage Review (DH, 2008b) and subsequent Transforming Community Services Programme (DH, 2009) established a framework to support new and existing social enterprises. NHS workers were also given the right to set up their own social enterprises through the 'Right to Request'. This provided English community health workers the opportunity to 'spin out' their services as a social enterprise, and successful applicants were to be awarded an initial contract to provide services for three to five years (DH, 2009; Miller and Lyon, 2016). The subsequent 'Right to Provide' programme (DH, 2011a) extended this right to all health and social care staff, although without the guarantee of contracts. New and existing social enterprises in health and social care were supported through the £120 million Social Enterprise Investment Fund (Hall et al, 2012a). The Any Qualified Provider policy has further opened up the NHS to private and third sector providers (DH, 2011b).

The implementation of the Social Value Act in 2013 gave further impetus to social enterprises. The Act requires commissioners of public services to 'consider how the services they commission and procure might improve the economic, social and environmental well-being of the area' (SEUK, 2012). Concepts such as 'happiness', 'well-being' and 'empowerment' are increasingly to be considered by public sector authorities when commissioning services (NAVCA, 2013). Research by the New Economics Foundation for the National Programme for Third Sector Commissioning provided evidence that commissioning from social enterprises and the broader third sector can capture the social, economic and environmental benefits that contribute to social value (Boyle and Murphy, 2009).

As a result of this conducive context, the third sector plays a significant role in the delivery of public services, including health and social care. The sector delivers around £7.2 billion or 17% of all social care, with the remainder being delivered 75% by the private sector and 8% by the public sector (Dickinson et al, 2012). Reprising the themes of the previous chapter, the third sector is said to be able to offer 'distinctive' welfare services that offer added value (Dickinson et al, 2012; Macmillan, 2013).

Micro-enterprise

Micro-enterprises are very small organisations that are usually defined by their number of employees. Like social enterprise, the term micro-enterprise lacks a fixed definition and the size of a micro-enterprise can vary considerably (MacGillivray et al, 2001; Fiedler, 2007; Pattie and Johnston, 2011). Related terms include micro-organisations (for example, Donahue, 2011) and micro-businesses (Matlay, 1999). Donahue's (2011) definition of micro-organisations is those with one or no paid employees, while the European Union refers to micro-enterprises as having fewer than 10 staff (FTE) and an annual turnover and/or annual balance sheet total that does not exceed €2 million (EU Recommendation 2003/361/EC, cited in Europa, 2003). According to a government-commissioned report (BIS, 2013), 95% of all businesses in the UK are micro-enterprises (defined as having fewer than 10 employees). These account for 32% of private sector employment.

The business models used by micro-enterprises vary widely; there is no set legal status or governance structure. A report by the micro-enterprise support organisation Community Catalysts (2011) indicates that micro-enterprises vary on a continuum from fully commercial at one end to fully voluntary at the other. The same report also shows that around 30–40% operate on a voluntary/semi-voluntary basis, while only some of the providers run a formally constituted business. Donahue (2011) adds that micro-organisations often have informal management structures that may resemble co-operatives in terms of decision making, roles and responsibilities, while Fox (2013) refers to micro-enterprises as often having mutual ownership. Although the term micro-enterprise is often associated (and even used interchangeably) with social enterprise (see, for example, Social Enterprise Academy, 2013), Lockwood (2013) states that micro-enterprises are not normally social enterprises, with only 10% of micro-enterprises meeting the criteria for a social enterprise, with the rest being established on a charity basis or a more conventional for-profit basis.

The wide variation in the legal status and structure of micro-enterprises therefore makes it difficult to define a 'micro-enterprise sector'. In fact, Lockwood (2013) found that the strategies designed to engage and support social enterprises more broadly, including start-up grants and training, are often unsuccessful with micro-enterprises. There has been criticism of the extent to which a rhetorical commitment by government to small-scale provision is borne out in local authority procurement and regulation policies (McCabe and Phillimore, 2012). Small and voluntary sector organisations compete with large, private sector providers and may not have the capacity to tender for contracts or to meet procurement criteria (DH and NAAPS, 2009; Rees, 2014). Local authorities, tasked with market development, may also lack the skills to undertake this role and it may conflict with other priorities, such as streamlining contracting procedures (Needham and Tizard, 2010).

Micro care providers

In the social care policy literature, micro-enterprises are usually defined as very small local enterprises with five or fewer paid or unpaid workers, set up to meet the needs of an individual or small group and being independent of any other organisation. This is the definition of micro-enterprises developed by Shared Lives Plus and Community Catalysts and used in publications by the DH and Think Local, Act Personal (DH and NAAPS, 2009; Community Catalysts, 2011, 2014; TLAP, 2011), and the definition we used in our study. This definition of micro-enterprise is smaller than that of a micro-business as set out above. It is bigger than the definition of a micro-organisation in the charitable sector, which is to have an annual turnover of less than £10,000 (likely to mean no paid staff at all) (NCVO, 2015). The definition does not include personal assistants (that is, care workers who support only one person): it applies to individuals or organisations providing services to two or more people.

We opted to use this definition for care-related micro-enterprise as a way of maximising the policy relevance of the research, and also because of its fit with the size profile of the sector. The NCVO definition is too small, given that we are looking at organisations that charge for their service, many of which will employ some staff. The EU threshold of 10 staff for a micro-business would be too big for the care sector, incorporating a wide range of established care organisations. Skills for Care data demonstrates the shape of the sector, with 46% of providers having fewer than 10 FTE staff (Skills for Care, 2015, p 13). By limiting the focus to five or fewer FTE, this still includes a high proportion of the sector. Skills for Care's size bandings do not map exactly onto ours, but its estimate that almost a third of the sector (31%) fit into the category of having 0–4 FTE staff highlights the dominance of very small organisations in the sector.

Micro-providers of care have been seen as particularly appropriate for a context of personal budgets for care service users, because the scale of provision matches the scale of commissioning (NHS Confederation, 2012). Whereas a local authority may struggle to commission multiple small contracts, an individual service user would have to deal with only one organisation. There has been considerable support from the DH for micro care provision. In the foreword to a DH–commissioned study on micro-enterprise, the then Minister of State for Care Services, Phil Hope, argued that 'The Department of Health sees micro-enterprises as vital elements of a diverse market that provides real choice to people' (DH and NAAPS, 2009, p 2).

Features of the sector, according to its exponents, are that micro-enterprises are offered by a range of people and organisations in the community, including by people who are disabled or who themselves need some support. These organisations may be run out of people's homes and employ members of extended family (Lockwood, 2013). Moreover, they may be motivated by a wish to help out a neighbour or friend rather than as a conventional social care business (DH and NAAPS, 2009). The support may also be delivered on an occasional basis, according to the needs of those they support, and also to fit in with other employment, personal caring responsibilities or study (DH and NAAPS, 2009). They therefore, arguably, bridge the third and fourth sectors, with the 'fourth sector' encompassing informal neighbourhood and community-based services that rely on informal local networks such as befriending and home visits by members of a church group (Williams, 2003; Hardill and Dwyer, 2011).

A definition of micro-enterprise by Lockwood (2013, p 27) highlights this distinctiveness, but also echoes the normative tone of much of the literature:

> Micro-providers are simply local people using their gifts and skills creatively to deliver support and services that benefit other local people and their community. They work on a very small scale, typically delivering their service directly with the help of a small number of other people working as employed staff or volunteers. They blur the distinction between service provider and service user – many people delivering micro-services themselves use social care and health services.

Such organisations do not necessarily fit well into a service and commissioning landscape that is used to larger and more formal organisations. It has been argued that well-tailored support for micro-enterprises, including start-up grants and training, as well as general information and advice, is very limited and often absent entirely (DH and NAAPS, 2009). Furthermore, any training in the social care sector may be expensive and/or focused on traditional provision so unsuitable for micro-enterprises (DH and NAAPS, 2009). In addition, micro-enterprises face challenges when it comes to business and IT expertise, as well as marketing skills, which makes it difficult for them to identify gaps in the market and for service users to find them (NAAPS, 2008; Doncaster Council, 2011). As stated in a foreword to a DH document (DH and NAAPS, 2009, p 3): 'Commissioners need to understand and support the conditions which make for healthy small organisations in order to provide a full range of choice and opportunity. This is particularly important with the advent of Personalisation, as many people needing support will choose micro organisations or personal assistants.'

Furthermore, regulation and legislative practices may not be set up with micro-enterprises in mind. Compliance processes around care, including for example CQC registration, are the same across the sector regardless of size (DH and NAAPS, 2009). Some commissioners and care managers may see non-traditional providers of care as more risky, and so restrict contracts to larger providers (NAAPS, 2008; DH and NAAPS, 2009). Small and voluntary organisations may also be ruled out of any tendering processes, as commissioners require certain levels of public liability insurance, or for organisations to have a minimum financial turnover (Valios, 2007). The contracts that are available to micro-enterprises are usually short term or piecemeal (less than a year), which leaves them with a constant struggle for income and unable to plan ahead (Dickinson et al, 2012). Insecure funding can also result in threats to care, due to staff insecurity leading to a high staff turnover and low morale (Cunningham and James, 2007; Dickinson et al, 2012). Micro-enterprises may also be unaware of funding opportunities or the capacity and business skills required to respond to tenders, or may be unable to understand funders' priorities and eligibility criteria (McCabe et al, 2010). Practical difficulties also arise around accessing insurance, Disability and Barring Service checks, policies and procedures (such as health and safety). Donahue (2011) argues that micro-organisations face a 'liability of smallness' in terms of their sustainability, legitimacy, volatility and operating environment. In such small organisations there is often an over-reliance on one individual (often the founder), who is heavily supported by informal networks.

Within micro-businesses of all kinds, there is known to be a high level of churn, a feature that has been intensified since 2008 by the recession (NCVO, 2011; Dellot, 2015). Research by the New Economics Foundation found that the majority of micro-entrepreneurs run their enterprise sub-legally and last about 18 months (MacGillivray et al, 2001). A report by the Department of Business, Industry and Skills (BIS, 2010) suggests that 90% of micro-enterprise start-ups fail within the first year (cited in Lockwood, 2013). Within the care sector, increased barriers around regulation, legislation and commissioning practices may also have led to a fall in the number of micro-enterprises (NAAPS, 2008). The DH funded a three-year project in collaboration with NAAPS (a membership organisation that supports providers of very small family- and community-based services) to stimulate the micro-enterprise market (DH and NAAPS, 2009). This work has been developed by Community Catalysts, an umbrella body set up to encourage micro-enterprises, who support around 600 micro-enterprises offering care and support services in the UK (Shared Lives Plus, 2011). It employs micro-enterprise coordinators in many areas around the country – people who actively support the development and sustainability of micro-enterprises in their locality. Evidence from Community Catalysts suggests that a local micro-enterprise coordinator decreases the rate of micro-enterprise failure from 90% per annum to 17% over three years (Shared Lives Plus, 2011).

Scaling up?

The previous chapter highlighted the extent to which size can be a dynamic state, with organisations shifting in size over time. In a working paper on scaling up social enterprise, Lyon and Fernandez (2012) note that 'there is considerable expectation placed on these types of organisations to have a larger scale of impact' and that many social enterprises have ambitions to grow. McCabe and Phillimore (2012) suggest that the trend towards fewer and larger contracts in the third sector has further encouraged organisational growth and mergers.

The focus on growth draws attention to the issue of how far all micro-enterprises should be seen as poised between growth or collapse, or whether 'micro' can be a sustainable size category. The high failure rate for micro-businesses suggests a context in which organisations that do not grow may be assumed to be on the verge of failure. Some of the third sector and social enterprise literature assumes that scaling up is the desired trajectory for all non-profits, conveying a sense that not to do so is socially harmful: 'The inability to achieve scale – that is, to make a meaningful and sustainable impact by reaching greater numbers of people – has limited the potential of these organizations and the people and causes they serve. Simply put, society's complex and pressing challenges call for solutions with a greater scale of impact' (Clark et al, 2012, p 1).

Indeed some sector leaders have decried the excessive smallness of too many organisations: According to the head of the Association of Chief Executives of the Voluntary Sector (ACEVO), Stephen Bubb: 'the sector is the wrong shape to make maximum use of the limited resources it is able to draw on: having a multitude of small organisations duplicating one another's work is not a good use of what capacity does exist in the sector. So we need to encourage more partnership working, more sharing of back-office facilities, and more mergers' (Bubb and Michell, 2009, p 76).

Strategies for organisational growth can include 'differentiation of services ..., diversification ..., increased market penetration, and growth through multiple sites' (Lyon and Fernandez, 2012). Scaling can also occur through franchising, or through less formal means such as training and membership networks (Lyon and Fernandez, 2012). However, the literature on growth has come to have more nuance, with increased discussion of non-replication scaling (Leat, 2003; Clark et al, 2012). As Clark et al explain:

in the last decade or so, the literature has shifted to include a broader definition of scale – moving away from the concept of scaling as organizational growth and towards the concept of scaling impact, or the outcomes the organization has generated beyond just the organization itself … A key distinction that has emerged in the literature is between strategies that involve *geographic replication* (for example, opening up new branches in order to implement a program model for new sets of beneficiaries) vs. what we call *non-replication options* (affiliating with new partners, disseminating ideas about change models directly or indirectly, working to change policy environments, and other strategies to create thought change or promote a social movement, etc. (Clark et al, 2012, p 5, emphasis in original)

This approach to growth can be seen in the work of the micro-enterprise support organisation Community Catalysts, which has focused on 'scaling out' through supporting a critical mass of such enterprises in localities rather than on encouraging scaling up of individual organisations (NHS Confederation, 2012).

A number of studies of very small organisations have made the point that such bodies are often happy to remain operating at a micro scale. In interviews with 'below the radar' groups and related policy makers, McCabe and Phillimore (2012) found little appetite for scaling up as a way to ameliorate increasingly adverse financial circumstances. A Putting People First-commissioned report on micro social care and support services makes the same point:

> Most providers of micro services are happy to provide services on a very small scale. This may be because they are committed to supporting one or two individuals; because they believe they can better retain control of their enterprise if it remains small; because they equate small scale with high quality and user led or because they want to work from home and in their community. The majority are not aiming to develop their enterprise in order to support more people or to expand into a different area. (DH and NAAPS, 2009, p 12)

Such claims suggest, then, that the extent to which organisations want to grow differs between sectors and is something to be alert to when researching micro-enterprises. It is a theme we return to in Chapter

Nine in exploring attitudes to growth within the organisations in our research study.

Four hypotheses about micro-enterprises

The aspiration to deliver services at a human scale that emerges from the personalisation reforms has led to a policy environment that is discursively supportive of delivering care and support through micro-enterprises. Such enterprises, with their low staff numbers, arguably approach the organisational embodiment of the human scale. Existing policy literature (often normative in tone) suggests that micro-enterprises have four benefits when compared to larger providers: they deliver more valued outcomes for the people being supported; they provide value for money; they are more personalised; and they are more innovative. Since micro care providers have received little academic attention, and the broader size, performance and innovation literatures discussed in Chapter Two was inconclusive, we have used the policy hypotheses as the starting point for the research. These four purported benefits are discussed in turn as the basis for generating hypotheses that are tested in the data:

Valued outcomes

The first perceived benefit is that micro-enterprises offer more valued outcomes for the people receiving support, when compared to larger providers. As Community Catalysts, the micro-enterprise support organisation, puts it, 'What do micro providers offer commissioners? Choice of tailored high quality local support and services for publically funded and self funded people – positive impact on well being and outcomes' (Community Catalysts, no date). The sorts of outcomes that the DH argues may be improved through being supported by micro-enterprises are diverse and include 'a reduction in the use of temporary accommodation, stronger communities, adult health and wellbeing, economic regeneration, job creation, tackling exclusion and promoting equality' (DH and NAAPS, 2009, p 20). They can also do this by drawing on local resources, which, for example, might include a micro-enterprise service operating from or holding meetings in a community café or social enterprise (Lockwood, 2013). Fox (2013) argues that by making people better connected, micro-enterprises can create social cohesion and tackle loneliness – issues that traditional care services don't tend to address. Examples support all of these claims, although not independent evaluation.

It is argued that micro-enterprises also support the delivery of the Social Value Act, requiring commissioners of public services to consider how the services they commission and procure might improve the economic, social and environmental well-being of the area (SEUK, 2012). In this sense micro-enterprises can be seen as contributing to the broader co-production agenda within public service (Needham and Carr, 2009; Durose et al, 2015). While co-production has been a thread of policy making in the care sector for a decade, the Care Act 2014 further formalised this, requiring local authorities to actively promote interventions that are co-produced with individuals, families, friends, carers and the community.

> H1: Micro-enterprises deliver more **valued outcomes** for users than larger organisations.

Cost-effective

The second claim made about micro-enterprises is that they are a cost-effective way to deliver care. This is a challenge to the economies-of-scale argument that has been one reason for the consolidation of much home and residential care into larger-scale units. As Lewis and West (2014, p 5) explain:

> local authorities largely abandoned spot contracts to meet the needs of a particular older person in favour of block contracts for 'set list' services, which worked out cheaper … outsourcing social care did save money. By 2009/10 the average unit cost of (usually more specialised) in-house local authority home care was £30.85p per hour, whereas the average cost for independent providers was £15.10p.

However, advocates of micro-enterprises have argued that such reasoning does not hold for very small providers and that highly specialised services can be delivered at a low cost: 'Micro-enterprises can often offer lower cost services, particularly when a highly tailored solution is desired, because they have few management and overhead costs' (NHS Confederation, 2012, p 5). They can mix paid and unpaid support to create a 'networked model of care' (Fox, 2013) that includes the informal support of family and friends, volunteers, paid carers and other professionals and services.

H2: Micro-enterprises **deliver more cost-effective outcomes** than larger organisations.

Personalised

The DH/NAAPS report sets out the claim that micro-enterprises are more person-centred:

> Tiny care and support services are able to help people in ways that are flexible, responsive and individual, making their services very attractive to service users and their families … They are local people providing local services to other local people. These providers support small numbers of people and this enables the provider to get to know the people who use the service, their family and supporters very well. (DH and NAAPS, 2009, p 8)

This approach offers a clear contrast to the 'time and task' model of care, in which highly specified and standardised services are provided, often by large organisations with high staff turnover (Burstow, 2014; Lewis and West, 2014). Instead, 'Micro-enterprises established and managed by local people are in a good position to deliver individualised services to people living in the same community … The service can offer consistency and genuine empathy and will often "stick with people" through difficult times' (DH and NAAPS, 2009, pp 4, 8). They are seen to be firmly rooted within a local community and so can have a good understanding of local needs and issues. As Donahue (2011, p 393), writing about micro-organisations more generally, states:

> Micro organisations can identify key needs within communities because they are run by people within those communities who have an organic understanding of the community, its problems and how best to address them.

They are seen to be able to provide more responsive and personal alternatives to mainstream activities and services, allowing them to engage with those who are most excluded (Donahue, 2011). They can also act as an intermediary by linking excluded groups with mainstream services that they may not otherwise access (Donahue, 2011).

H3: Micro-enterprises are better than larger organisations at delivering services that **are personalised to the individual**.

Innovative

A fourth claim made about micro-enterprises is that they are likely to be more innovative than large providers, since they work closely with users and can respond in a flexible way to user demand (DH and NAAPS, 2009; DH, 2010). This stems from the idea that the informal and often fluid nature of micro-enterprises means that most may look nothing like traditional health and social care services (Lockwood, 2013), thereby making them more creative and flexible. As stated by the DH (2010, p 8):

> The entrepreneurialism, innovation, creativity and pioneering approach of very small providers can offer a great deal to the wider social care sector by giving a clear demonstration to local authorities and larger providers of what can be achieved in response to the personalisation agenda.

Micro-enterprises may therefore be able to offer alternative solutions to social care needs within a diversified care market.

Innovation can also arise as a result of working in different ways with citizens and service users. Within the public sector especially, there has been a realisation that innovation can occur by making use of capacity outside of existing organisations by 'empowering communities' and devolving power, choice and control to front-line professionals and the public (LGA/Locality, 2012). This can include involving 'seldom heard' communities, marginalised from mainstream services, linked to ethnic or sexual identities (Needham and Carr, 2015). Users and consumers of services, as well as other citizens, can contribute to innovation in public services as partners in designing and delivering services (Harris and Albury, 2009, p 2). This further supports the drive towards co-production discussed above.

H4: Micro-enterprises are more **innovative** than larger organisations.

These four claims have been derived from reports that have significant input or authorship from organisations that support micro-enterprise development and are based on a small number of case studies. There has been a lack of independent evaluation of micro-enterprises, or of research that compares micro-enterprises with larger providers, in the way that we do here.

Conclusion

This chapter began by situating micro-enterprises within the broader context of public service reform, which, beginning in the 1990s, has seen radical shifts in social care and other welfare services. Within social care, services that were previously provided by local authorities are now being delivered by a range of non-governmental providers. As a result, the private sector now delivers around three-quarters of all social care. The third sector, including small community services, also plays a key role in the delivery of social care, especially for non-traditional or marginalised service users. Recent government policy has sought to further extend and diversify the social care market, looking to increase the supply of social enterprises.

The Care Act 2014 calls for a diversification of the social care market that includes more user-led organisations and small businesses. In addition to increasing the supply of micro-enterprises, policy levers associated with the personalisation agenda are expected to increase the demand for such services. This includes the introduction of personal budgets, which devolve some financial control to individuals who use services. Policy has also sought to raise demand for micro-enterprises from commissioners, through, for example, the Social Value Act, which requires commissioners of public services, including social care, to purchase services from providers who deliver added social value. However, barriers remain in place, associated with procurement and regulation.

This chapter and the previous one have set out the policy context in which micro-enterprises operate. Four hypotheses have been set out for testing, based on policy literature that has often had an explicitly normative thrust. The next two chapters deal with aspects of methodology before we move on to the findings from the research project in Chapter Six and subsequent chapters.

FOUR

Methods for co-productive research

There are (at least) two ways to tell the story about research methods. The first is to present it as a neat flow of what was done, to how many people and how the resultant data was analysed. However, there is an alternative story, one that is much more messy and problematic, of organisations that did not fit into the size boundaries that we had established for micro, small, medium and large providers; of clashing norms of research between community researchers and academic researchers. In this chapter and the next we offer a bit of both. We provide the broad outline of how we did the research, who we spoke to, what data collection and analysis processes were involved and the participatory approach we took to involve people with experience of care services as co-researchers. We also discuss the ways in which the research changed as a result of unexpected practices and dilemmas presented when we left our desks for the case study sites. In the next chapter we discuss how we sampled the 27 organisations which took part in the study.

The research took a co-produced approach, involving people with experience of using and delivering services as co-researchers in the project. Patient and service user research involvement is becoming more embedded into the health and social care system as part of a broader ethical commitment to research as a co-productive process (Durose et al, 2015; Flinders et al, 2015). There is a growing consensus around the need to develop a more rigorous approach to understanding the impact of service user researchers – one that challenges all involved to reconnect with the potential of what can be gained and to recognise why service users are being included (Roy, 2012; INVOLVE, 2013). The benefits of involving service users as researchers, such as increasing individuals' skills, strengthening communities and gaining relevant insights for service change, have become strong themes reinforced within national policy and, as such, are often taken for granted (Flinders et al, 2015). This chapter outlines the study's methodological approach and discusses how taking a co-productive approach changed the research process. Drawing on the study's experience of training and researching alongside people with experience of local care services, the chapter makes links to current debates about participatory approaches and practices.

Research design

As set out in Chapter Three, four testable hypotheses drawn from the policy literature formed the basis of our approach to the research design.

H1 Micro-enterprises deliver more **valued outcomes** for users than larger organisations.

H2 Micro-enterprises deliver more **cost-effective** outcomes than larger organisations.

H3 Micro-enterprises are better than larger organisations at delivering services that are **personalised** to the individual.

H4 Micro-enterprises are more **innovative** than larger organisations.

Qualitative interviews and ASCOT survey questions formed the central methods for collecting data. Interviews undertaken with staff, service users and carers were designed to provide insight into all four hypotheses. Data collected through ASCOT was specifically designed to analyse the first two hypotheses: (1) to calculate outcome scores for service users and carers and (2) to assess value for money by comparing outcome scores with pricing data gathered during the interviews. There was a significant difference between how we originally envisaged undertaking the interviews and using ASCOT and how we eventually chose to apply these methods. Our changes were the result of piloting and of co-researcher involvement, discussed in more detail below. The first part of the chapter considers the contribution of co-researchers to the project – discussing their involvement, the ways that this shaped the research project and the findings from the evaluation that came at the end of the project. The second half of the chapter addresses other aspects of methodology, including research ethics, recruitment of interviewees and data analysis.

The co-production approach

Undertaking the research with local co-researchers opened us up to the practice that Wagenaar stipulates as key to effective research: '*Organise your research in such a way that you create the conditions for surprise*' (Wagenaar, 2011, p 243, emphasis in the original). In other words, by including the original perspectives of co-researchers with experience of local care services we sought in part to inject something novel into the research process and, in doing so, to provide more relevant and valid findings.

There are increasing attempts to consolidate learning into overarching strategies and practical guidance for involving service users as researchers (Beresford, 2007; SCIE, 2007; INVOLVE, 2013). The following are some of the strongest messages about how to involve service users.

- Co-researchers should be involved in *different stages* of the research process.
- An *individual approach* is required so that service users' unique skills can be recognised and in order to provide the effective support.
- Participative research should have clear and measurable *outcomes*.
- Research teams should appraise how co-researcher involvement *impacts* on the achievement of these outcomes.

These principles formed a guide for our overall approach to research design. Figure 4.1 shows the research activities undertaken by co-researchers and the related outcomes that were expected to improve the quality of the study. Involving co-researchers in as many different aspects of the research process as possible was an explicit aim. This was not simply an issue of maximising co-researchers' practical engagement with the research; it was part of a more fundamental shift, rebalancing decision-making power and ownership of the research. Rather than merely servicing research through data-collection roles, the study aimed to encourage co-researchers to have an active role in the interpretation and analysis of data and in communicating directly with research, health and social care audiences. Through this we aimed to align our approach with a wider concept of co-production in public services, where 'individuals, communities and organisations have the skills, knowledge and ability to work together, create opportunities and solve problems' (NDTI and Helen Sanderson Associates, 2010, p 3).

However, an aspect of the methodological 'messiness' described at the beginning of the chapter was that, despite our commitment to a co-productive approach at all stages, there were some research activities, especially in the early planning phase, that did not involve co-researchers. Due to the need to specify aspects of the research design in the original research council funding bid, we had to plan elements in advance of knowing where the three research localities would be (and we could not recruit the co-researchers in advance of that decision). Having received the research funding and identified the sites, we also needed to get approval from the national Social Care Research Ethics Committee before recruiting co-researchers in these localities. The ethical review process required that we should produce participant information sheets, consent forms and interview schedules and have

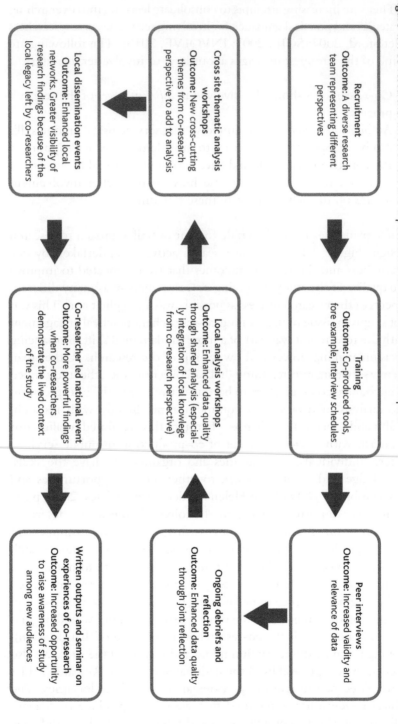

Figure 4.1: Co-researcher involvement and expectations for enhanced research outputs

Recruitment
Outcome: A diverse research team representing different perspectives

Training
Outcome: Co-produced tools, fore example, interview schedules

Cross site thematic analysis workshops
Outcome: New cross-cutting themes from co-research perspective to add to analysis

Local dissemination events
Outcome: Enhanced local networks. Greater visibility of research findings because of the local legacy left by co-researchers

Local analysis workshops
Outcome: Enhanced data quality through shared analysis (especially integration of local knowlege from co-research perspective)

Co-researcher led national event
Outcome: More powerful findings when co-researchers demonstrate the lived context of the study

Peer interviews
Outcome: Increased validity and relevance of data

Ongoing debriefs and reflection
Outcome: Enhanced data quality through joint reflection

Written outputs and seminar on experiences of co-research
Outcome: Increased opportunity to raise awareness of study among new audiences

a clear plan for how many co-researchers to recruit and what activities they would undertake, all of which was therefore pre-drafted before the process of co-researcher recruitment began. The literature review phases were also conducted before co-researcher involvement, as these took place while we were waiting for ethical approval.

Clearly, it is frustrating that so much of the project design pre-dated co-researcher involvement. While this was largely out of our control, lessons learned from this study have helped us to identify two ways to mitigate these factors: the first is that we now have an established team of co-researchers in three parts of the country that we are hoping to work with on future projects and – given our established links – we can involve them at the beginning of research design rather than only after many aspects of the design have solidified. Second, we would in future seek to persuade research funders and ethics committees of the benefits of leaving open certain aspects of the research design if co-researchers are to make a meaningful contribution to the design phase. This is, of course, difficult to achieve in practice: ethics committees want to be assured that co-researchers – drawn from populations considered 'vulnerable' (Brown, 2015) – are being involved in a viable and ethical research process. However, we would like to get support for some aspects of the research design to be left undeveloped until co-researchers join the project.

Recruiting, training and paying co-researchers

Co-researchers in the three localities were recruited through advertising in local care networks such as carers' newsletters, local authority employment services, local Age UK branches and Healthwatch. People interested in applying were asked to complete an application form and were then interviewed by us over the telephone. Eligibility was based on evidence of applicants meeting the person specification for the role. The people selected after this process were then asked to attend two days of training in their local area. The role of academic researchers as selectors of the co-researchers again underlines the explicit power disparities within this relationship.

Following good practice in user involvement, funding was available to pay the co-researchers for the time spent interviewing (NIHR, 2013), although we did not have funding available to pay co-researchers to attend the training. Expenses were provided for all activities on the project, including training sessions and paying for respite care arrangements for those family carers who became co-researchers. Box 4.1 displays the characteristics of the 20 co-researchers who took part in interviewing (three trained co-researchers did not undertake the interviews, due to care commitments or health issues).

Box 4.1: Co-researcher characteristics

Twenty people were recruited and trained as co-researchers.

Seventeen of these co-researchers undertook interviews.

Nine co-researchers were older people with care responsibilities.

Six co-researchers were people with autism or learning disabilities.

Two co-researchers were personal assistants to co-researchers with learning disabilities, and also had family care responsibilities.

Our original intention was to recruit people with learning disabilities, older people and informal carers. The inclusion of professional carers/ personal assistants as co-researchers came about through our initial meetings with people with learning disabilities. During the training two of the co-researchers with learning disabilities were accompanied by personal assistants (PAs). There were three aspects that led to the inclusion of these individuals as co-researchers. Firstly, their enthusiasm for the topic: the PAs joined in quite naturally during training sessions, offering valuable insights into care experience and local knowledge of the sector. Secondly, the research activity became something that the service user and their PA could do together, rather than the service user simply 'being supported'. The PAs did still support their clients to different extents, in one case just with transport (as that was all that was required) and in the second case by spending time to go over the training materials with the person to reassure her and refresh her engagement with the study. Lastly, both of the PAs had experience of informal care roles as well as being professional carers, again increasing their potential insights as co-researchers. We decided to offer them the opportunity to join the project as co-researchers who would undertake carer interviews.

The research team worked to identify when co-researchers were in receipt of benefits and to understand when payment could endanger those benefits. We found it really difficult to get reliable, accurate information about payments and benefits, which created anxieties for everyone involved. Advice from the Citizens Advice Bureau suggested that each person's situation would be different and that they needed one-to-one guidance, but in each locality there wasn't necessarily appropriate guidance available. Academic researchers worked through this in dialogue with co-researchers and their families. In at least one case a co-researcher with autism receiving Employment and Support Allowance couldn't find enough clear guidance about their permitted earnings and so decided not to get paid at all. This type of situation sends the wrong message to co-researchers about the value of their contribution, and is something we will strive to resolve in future projects.

The training was undertaken over two days in each of the three local sites, and run by the project team (a further reminder of the power dynamic in the academic researcher–co-researcher relationship). It was unpaid and it felt appropriate to invite people to give up only two full days for training, rather than to extend it over a longer period. However, this limited the amount of material that could be covered. The first day was spent encouraging the co-researchers to get to know each other and us, familiarising them with the research focus and generating ideas for potential interview questions that would allow testing of the four hypotheses. The second day was spent on interview techniques and role plays and how to troubleshoot potential problems that might come up in the interviews, such as how to get quieter people to say more, or how to bring people back to the topic. We also looked at how we would be arranging the practical aspects of the interviews, such as transport requirements of co-researchers.

Our approach to generating interview questions was to describe the main research areas that we wanted the interviews to focus on and then ask co-researchers to create questions in their own words, designed for their peers, that might tap into relevant information. Appendix 1, 'Site one interview schedule', displays the types of interview questions suggested by co-researchers in site one and captures how we presented the questions with additional prompts about introductions, taking consent, the ASCOT survey and thanking the interviewee. Ideas for interview questions were developed by co-researchers in three local sites. However, to ensure some level of similarity across the interviews we shared with sites two and three the previous interview questions devised by co-researchers in site one. Co-researchers often critiqued the other questions before producing their own versions. These minor variations are not expected to have a significant impact on interview responses or findings, as all questions remained rooted in understanding whether care services were valued, personalised, innovative and value for money.

Two aspects of our research design changed as a result of the training session and the early piloting of the work in site one. The first was that we adapted our use of ASCOT to make it better fit the interview setting. The second was that we shifted away from our original intention of using narrative interviewing and towards a more semi-structured approach.

Use of ASCOT

ASCOT is a validated outcomes tool used to measure an individual's social care-related quality of life (SCRQoL). The tool is used in national surveys by the DH and is designed to be applied across user groups and in different care settings. On these grounds ASCOT was a good methodological and practical match for our study. Not only would we be able to apply it across diverse services but it would also deliver standardised measures suitable for national comparative analysis.

Understanding the principles behind the survey, why we were planning to use it and how best to administer it to people who might have learning disabilities or dementia was not something that could be covered in the time available to train co-researchers. As academic researchers we had had two full days of training on ASCOT from the team who developed the tool at the University of Kent, and we could not replicate this as well as cover the other relevant material in the time we had available for co-researcher training. We felt that an appropriate compromise was for us to administer the ASCOT survey in the last section of the interview, after the co-researcher had asked the interview questions. This seemed consistent with an interpretation of co-research in which both people play a role in interviewing. The co-researcher would lead and run the main part of the interview, handing over briefly to the academic researcher for ASCOT, before the co-researcher wrapped up the interview.

There are a number of ASCOT tools available that can be used to generate data for measures of SCRQoL, such as self-completion questionnaires, interviews and observation tools. This study used the interview version (INT4) that measures four levels of need: ideal state, no needs, some needs and high needs. Using the INT4 tool allows researchers to measure the current and expected SCRQoL for each interviewee. Drawing on the data from the DH's Adult Social Care Survey, we were able to look at how the current SCRQoL of the participants differed from national averages.

However, we had to make further modifications to our use of ASCOT following a pilot phase of the research. We originally planned to administer all nine domains of the ASCOT survey, asking about the different domains and ranking the respondent's quality of life against the four scored outcome levels – a total of 23 questions. However, the ASCOT survey proved to be an awkward fit into the interviews. We had agreed in discussion with the co-researchers that ASCOT would come at the end of the interview, after the more discursive interview phase, given its more structured format and closed questions, which might close down questioning if used at the start of the interview. However, by the end of the interview people were tired and the full survey felt far too long to administer.

After piloting the full version, we decided to limit the ASCOT to two of its nine domains (choice and control; and how people spend their time), which were the most relevant for all the services and people included in the study. Other domains – for example those relating to people's personal cleanliness or to food and drink preparation – were not appropriate to some of the services in our sample. The ASCOT team at the University of Kent provided confirmation that the tool could be used in this modified form. With only two domains we were unable to calculate an overall SCRQoL, but we could still undertake the national comparison, since the national data can be disaggregated into the separate domains. Appendix 2 displays the two-domain version of ASCOT that we used.

With this adaptation, the interviews in practice were shorter than we had planned. We had anticipated that they would take two hours, to allow time for introductions, taking consent, the narrative phase and the full ASCOT survey. However, in practice the maximum length was an hour and some were shorter. Interviewees in the pilot interviews looked alarmed that we might take two hours (even though this had been mentioned in advanced) and we quickly learned that an hour was a time span that participants felt much more comfortable with and that felt appropriate for everyone's energy levels. The shorter version of ASCOT made it possible to cover the material in an hour. Most of the interviews with people who use a micro-enterprise for support in the home took the full hour or longer. People were heavily invested in the service and had a lot to say about it. Some of the other types of micro service, for example drama groups and football sessions, were smaller (though valued) parts of people's lives and service experiences were relayed within a shorter time.

From narrative to semi-structured interviewing

An implication of working with co-researchers, which was not evident to us until we undertook pilot interviews, was that we needed extra time in the training to explain what we meant by narrative approaches to interviewing, and why we considered it to be a worthwhile approach. Following Riessman (1993, 2001) and Wengraf (2001), we had planned to use a narrative approach to interviewing, in recognition that individuals' experience of care services is constructed as part of their wider life story and identity. The intention of the research had been to capture people's genuine and felt experience of services, with the co-researchers encouraging the interviewees to speak freely and at length. Our assumption was that this would be an intuitive style of interviewing for service user researchers that didn't require much training. As Greenhalgh et al put it, 'In narrative interview the researcher invites participants to "tell me what happened" and allows them to speak uninterrupted until the story ends ... prompts should only be used to preserve the flow of the story' (Greenhalgh et al, 2005, p 444).

That there is a craft to this, rather than its being an intuitive conversation style, was something that we became much more strongly aware of during the project. In pilot interviews, the co-researchers were more comfortable working through the questions on the interview guide as a series of semi-structured questions, rather than as prompts for a narrative flow. This meant that in many cases the interviews followed a question–and–response format rather than being a story-telling encounter. For the co-researchers, having spent time developing the questions, there was an assumption that an interview was a process of working through them in order. This sometimes meant asking an interviewee a question that had already been covered in a previous response. The practice of working dynamically with a set of prompts while also listening to someone's talk is something we had experience of from our PhD research and subsequent projects. We failed to appreciate the need to train more explicitly in that skill, and the amount of training time we had available did not make this possible.

We may indeed have made the problem worse in the training by highlighting the problem of irrelevant material, getting co-researchers to role-play how to get people back on track if they wandered off the target. As a result some co-researchers felt that they were failing if they did not keep the interview tightly focused on answering the questions. Wagenaar warns:

> Inexperienced interviewers sometimes express reluctance to let the respondent explore his observations and experiences ... because they are afraid they might get richly detailed but irrelevant material. It is often difficult to arrange an interview and you run the risk of blowing your one chance if the respondent goes off at a tangent. Better to follow a strict protocol of questions, then. Underlying this remark is a deep-seated urge to control the interview because it might deviate from the question or theory that animated the project. (Wagenaar, 2011, p 258)

Wagenaar's comments are directed at inexperienced academic researchers, but we felt that this was also evident in the co-researchers' engagement with the interview experience. It highlighted for us the need to use training to develop familiarity with the use of prompt tools, especially when working with people who lack confidence in their own ability to communicate.

This insight is also relevant to the people being interviewed, as well as for the interviewer. Some interviewees' capacity and confidence for telling stories may also have made narrative responses more difficult to achieve. Many respondents with learning disabilities seemed to prefer giving shorter answers. The passage below shows part of an interview between two people with learning disabilities.

> *Co-researcher:* Right, [interviewee name]. I'm going to start asking you, by asking you a few questions. How did you find out about this service? Like football, how did you find out about this football?
> *Respondent:* By [name of the person who runs the service]
> *Co-researcher:* Is the service user-friendly?
> *Respondent:* Yeah.
> *Co-researcher:* Can you get in touch with [the person who runs the service] out of hours, so after the football?
> *Respondent:* Yeah.
> *Co-researcher:* Are you happy with the service?
> *Respondent:* Yeah.
> *Co-researcher:* Does it meet your needs?
> *Respondent:* Yeah.
> *Co-researcher:* It does, good. Say you had a problem, would you be able to go to [him] about it?
> *Respondent:* Yeah.

> *Co-researcher:* Good. How do you pay for this service? Do you have an IB, an individual budget?
> *Respondent:* I just pay.
> *Co-researcher:* Or do you just pay out of your own, like spare money?
> *Respondent:* Pay out my money. (Person with learning disabilities 206, Micro day service)

As co-researchers got used to their interviewing roles we saw that they increasingly veered away from their 'scripts' in order to create a more relaxed exchange. For instance, instead of asking, 'Does the service meet your needs?', one co-researcher asked, 'What about the activities here, do you like 'em? Do they fit with what you want, what you like doing?'

Our interviews, then, were not narrative interviews – which is not to say, of course, that the responses were not storied. If narrative is taken in Bruner's (1986) sense of the 'science of the imagination', with its focus on understanding specific phenomena in terms of 'human experience and purpose', then narratives remain central to the work.

Evaluating co-researcher involvement

In addition to our own real-time adaptations of the research design to make it work better as a co-researched process, the study incorporated an evaluation of co-researcher involvement, undertaken by two colleagues who had not been directly involved in other stages of the research process (Littlechild and Tanner, 2015). The evaluation focused on how co-researchers undertook activities; the role of the academic researchers; and what factors helped or hindered the co-production of research. The following three methods were used to evaluate the co-researcher involvement.

- Conversation analysis of a sample of 18 interviews undertaken by co-researchers across the three sites.
- Three focus groups with 15 of the co-researchers, one in each of the research sites, asking them about their experiences of involvement in the research project.
- Individual face-to-face semi-structured interviews with the three academic researchers, asking about their rationale for the research model and their experiences of working with co-researchers.

The evaluation identified two key aspects of co-researcher involvement that have also been recognised in broader literature on peer research. The first was the extent to which co-researchers established a rapport with the people they were interviewing; the second was about the training and support that was provided to the co-researchers. Key findings from the evaluation are presented here. A summary of the evaluation is available (Littlechild and Tanner, 2015) and a fuller discussion will be published in the future.

Establishing rapport

INVOLVE's (2013) exploration of the impact of public involvement on the quality of research highlights data collection as one of six main areas for positive impact. Cook, a researcher working with people with neurological conditions, explained that these in-depth discussions often happened because people with experience asked more 'direct and searching questions' and because it matters to the participant that the interviewer has similar personal experience. As a result, participants often express very personal ideas and experiences, commenting 'that they had never shared certain information with anyone else' (INVOLVE, 2013, p 7).

However, one of the findings from our study was that broad categories such as 'older people' or 'people with learning disabilities' cover such a range of individuals that co-researchers did not always feel a connection. This was most pronounced for people with learning disabilities who were interviewing others with more profound disabilities, especially when the interviewees did not follow communication conventions such as facing the interviewer or had very limited verbal capacity. In post-interview debriefs co-researchers described the interviews as "draining", "uncomfortable", "needing to be patient" and spoke about not knowing what to do and "clamming up". This gives an insight into the limitations of peer interviewing and the danger of assuming shared characteristics or empathy within very broad categories.

Many co-researchers did demonstrate a high level of skill in teasing out information and also used their shared experiences to forge a relationship with participants. The following quotations from the evaluation focus groups indicate this.

> "Due to having a disability myself I found it easier to link with some of the people and they felt more at ease. And having the knowledge and used some of the services was

easy to relate to their experiences." (Co-researcher with learning disabilities, Evaluation focus group)

Another co-researcher talked about the characteristics that she thought made a difference:

"Our age and our personality, you know, our empathy, our background, all sorts of things and I think the people who do this work really need to be the right people." (Co-researcher, carer, Evaluation focus group)

One co-researcher recognised that to put participants at ease, the shared experience does not have to be about services. It could simply be a shared accent and familiarity with the area.

"It does help if you know the area and if you can speak in the local vernacular, you know, and say 'how bin ya?' I wouldn't say that but ... if you can use that accent or I say 'yeah, I know that chip shop down the road'." (Co-researcher, carer, Evaluation focus group)

The relaxed atmosphere created by the presence of co-researchers could put the academic researcher at ease, as well as the participant. The following account from one of the academic researchers shows the value of the co-researcher having previous volunteering experience rather than shared experience.

"In one case we went to see to see a man who had a range of health problems, lived in quite squalid accommodation and when we went in he didn't have any trousers on, just covered by a towel and I think I would have found that a quite difficult setting on my own but [name of co-researcher] who I was with who'd been an Age UK volunteer, I got the impression he wasn't fazed by it, or certainly didn't show it. Just got on and settled down. In a setting like this it was really helpful to have him there." (Academic researcher, Evaluation interview)

Overall, the evaluation found clear benefits from co-researchers sharing key characteristics with participants. This was recognised in relation to the positive atmosphere created in interviews and the discussions of mutual experience of local service issues that the academic researcher may not have been aware of. However, the evaluation did identify some co-researchers who did not see their shared experience as enhancing the interviews, and this leads to two key observations. Firstly, it reflects the conclusion of several critical commentaries (McLaughlin, 2009; Roy, 2012), highlighting that the participation of services users in and of itself will not always lead to enhanced research practice. Secondly, it signals that the benefits of shared experience may be fully realised only if it is acknowledged and reflected upon explicitly as an important part of the training and design of interviews. While some co-researchers knew how to use their shared experience as helpful in the interview setting, others may have benefited from being able to reflect on this and learn from their fellow co-researchers.

Coaching and development

The evaluation captured the shared view of both co-researchers and academic researchers about the need to improve the training. There were mixed views about whether the amount of time was right or not, but an overall consensus that more interactive/practice work should be included, with additional individual coaching where people felt it would help them build confidence in the role. There was also agreement that the training should cover different areas, such as how to interview people who communicate differently and more clarity about how to use prompt questions to achieve a narrative-style conversation. Preparation and debriefing sessions around the interviews were also seen as important. Co-researchers found their role easiest when they felt they knew exactly what was expected of them, and some found it reassuring that the academic researcher could step in during the interview if they were struggling. Evaluators saw that where there was mutual understanding between the academic researcher and co-researcher, the interviews were more fluid and confident. The evaluation specifically pointed to the potential usefulness of individual coaching sessions (something that happened accidentally with one co-researcher with learning disabilities and their personal assistant and was found to be a useful exercise). As one co-researcher with learning disabilities commented about the training:

> "They should have done at least two weeks, not two days, because to learn something like that in two days just isn't – well particularly with disabled people, I think for a non-disabled probably yes but for disabled people I think it

needed to be a two week training session … to me." (Co-researcher with learning disabilities, Evaluation focus group)

The sorts of problems experienced in the co-research process seemed to focus on people's confidence in their role and self-awareness. In particular it felt important to know whom they might be interviewing and how to overcome difficulties.

Extending training sessions is one way to address these issues, although there may be practical limitations in terms of the time that co-researchers want to commit in advance of a project that they don't yet know if they will benefit from and enjoy: training needs to not be so long that potential co-researchers are put off from applying for the role. There may also be a role for greater ongoing open reflection in small groups. This might help to build all researchers' confidence in their role and actions, help to learn from each other and build a deeper engagement with the co-production of research. During the study there were several opportunities for such reflection both within sites and between academic and co-researcher; however, these tended to be part of other events, such as while travelling or as part of an analysis workshop. Creating dedicated time for this activity may be a better way to ensure that potential problems surface early and can be addressed.

Ethics

Formal ethical review of the study by the national Social Care Research Ethics Committee (SCREC) has already been mentioned in relation to our co-research approach. We were aware that, as a project which involved adults with an assessed social care need (as co-researchers and interviewees), our research required full ethical scrutiny. We set out for the SCREC our planned approach in relation to sampling, consent, information, confidentiality, scope to withdraw from the project and data management, drawing on broad ethical standards (for example, British Psychological Society, 2009) as well as comparable work with co-researchers (Ellins et al, 2012). Under guidance from SCREC we developed a safeguarding protocol to utilise if we had concerns that people taking part in the project were at risk of harm.

We had hoped to design a consent process that enabled the participation of people who were unable to give consent themselves, by identifying a partner, close friend or relative to act as a consultee in accordance with the Mental Capacity Act. We recognise that people who are unable to give informed consent may nonetheless be able to express their views and feelings about their situation and the services they use (Ellins et al, 2012). However, we were required by the SCREC to only include people who could give consent themselves.

The inclusion of co-researchers and participants with learning disabilities led the SCREC to request EasyRead versions of recruitment materials, consent forms and information sheets. We worked with a local social enterprise to develop resources that met the European EasyRead Standard. These EasyRead documents were well received by co-researchers and were especially useful for enabling co-researchers with learning disabilities to take the lead during the interviews in explaining key information about the project and taking consent.

The SCREC also highlighted anonymity of the interview participants and confidentiality of the data as a key issue in research design when working with small organisations and requested further assurance of how these would be protected. We acknowledged that it was possible that co-researchers and interviewees might know each other, particularly in settings where there were a small number of learning disability services that they both might access. We agreed to inform the co-researcher and the interviewee of each other's names prior to the interview and ask both to highlight if there was any conflict of interest or if they are unhappy to proceed. We also made sure that the importance of confidentiality was reinforced in each training session and at the start and end of every interview. To comply with SCREC requirements in relation to anonymity, we did not name the three localities in which we undertook the research; the Committee felt that the distinctive features of micro-enterprises were such that their identity could be worked out from the locality even if we did not name any organisation or individual that took part.

Interviews

As discussed above, the interviews were guided by a schedule that was developed in collaboration with the co-researchers. The schedules were developed separately in each locality but all included discussion of why people had selected the care organisation, what relationships they had with staff, how much the provision was tailored to their needs and what they perceived to be the strengths and weaknesses of the service. In this way the interviews were designed to capture data about the value of services to their users, as well as capturing the personalised nature and extent of innovation evident in different care services. All participants were given an EasyRead information sheet about the project and asked to sign a consent form in advance of the interview starting. The research focused on staff, service users and

Table 4.1: Interviews and ASCOT surveys (*N*)

	Co-ordinators	Staff	Older people	People with disabilities	Carers	Total
Site 1: Urban local authority in the North West	2	9	0	27	9	47
Site 2: Two local authorities in the West Midlands with mixed urban and rural profile	2	13	7	20	11	53
Site 3: Rural county in the East Midlands	1	10	23	2	7	43
Total interviews	5	32	30	49	27	143
Total ASCOT survey completions			30	49	16	95

family carers in 27 organisations (a mix of micro, small, medium and large) in three localities. Sampling of these organisations is discussed in the next chapter.

A total of 143 interviews were undertaken for the project. This included 5 interviews with micro-coordinators (the people in the localities who had a role in developing micro care provision) and 32 interviews with staff members from each organisation, usually the manager and/or person who had set up the organisation. There were more than 27 because some organisations provided two interviewees. A further 106 interviews were with people who used services, and family carers. We had aimed for three users and one carer from all 27 organisations (totalling 108), but two interviewees dropped out and couldn't be replaced. All interviews were conducted face to face in the provider settings or the homes of service users. There were four exceptions to this where interviews were carried out over the phone, at the request of the interviewee. All interviews were audio-recorded and later transcribed.

Coordinator interviews focused on their role, the local micro-enterprise sector and other contextual local issues in relation to social care. Staff interview questions asked about why they had set up the organisation, what services they provided, how much they charged, what relationship they had with the local authority and what, if anything, they saw as distinctive in the support they provided. Staff and coordinator interviews were undertaken by a member of the academic research team. Interviews ended by researchers asking if the staff member would be willing to approach people using the service and carers so as to request their permission to be contacted by the research team. We left it to each organisation to select three respondents and a carer for us to interview. For many of the micro-enterprises, who had only a handful of clients, this meant contacting everyone they supported to see who would be willing to speak to us. The larger organisations could be more selective, and we recognise this as a limit of the sampling approach. However, we would have found it very difficult to get contact details of the people using the service other than by using this contact method. The people we interviewed from the larger organisations at times were critical about the services they received, so we had no reason to suspect that the organisations had offered interviews with only their 'happy customers'.

The 106 service users and carers were asked about their care provider, including why they had selected the care organisation, what relationships they had with staff, how much the provision was tailored to their needs and what they perceived to be the strengths and weaknesses of the service. They included 30 older people, 49 people with a learning disability (or impairment such as autism) and 27 carers. Participants in the interviews included a mix of self-funders and people funded by local authorities. At the end of each interview participants were asked questions from the two ASCOT domains. The ASCOT survey was completed by the 79 people who used services. Where carers were interviewed separately (in 16 cases) we also asked them to score the service on the ASCOT domains, bringing the total of completed surveys to 95.

In designing the research we had envisaged that we would be interviewing either a user or a carer singly, but in practice that was not always the case. Family carers often sat in on interviews with people who use services and the interviews were therefore multi-vocal experiences of people with different perspectives on common events. This caused some practical limitations and methodological issues. Co-researchers and academic researchers shared concerns that having others present would bias or limit the way that family carers and people who use services spoke about those services. However, we felt that we had limited scope in practice to ask people to leave the room when we were in their homes without damaging the rapport that interview-based research requires. Where family carers were present we ensured that we took consent from them as well as from the person using the care service.

Undertaking some of the interviews as multi-lateral conversations including people classed as 'carers' as well as those classed as 'users' underscored for us the problematic nature of these binary identities: 'This reification of roles within caring relationships obscures the complexity of individual identity and ignores the intersectionality of people's experience' (Barnes et al, 2015, p 15). We continue to use the labels here because they are a useful shorthand, and in part capture the nature of the caring relationships at the point in time when we did the interviews. However, we recognise here and elsewhere in the book that even so this is an over-simplification of the 'mutual interdependency' of many care relationships (Ward, 2015, p 167).

Analysis

Given the importance of a co-productive research design to our overall methodology, we took a twin-track approach to analysis. It was essential to find a balance between incorporating the perspective of co-researchers into the analysis and ensuring a systematic analysis of a large volume of interview transcripts. As a result, some analysis activities were undertaken by the academic team, for example analysing interview transcripts in QSR-NVivo and formulating cost-effectiveness data from ASCOT scores. Other activities were designed specifically to feed co-researcher interpretations into the analysis process.

Co-researchers' perspectives were incorporated through ongoing debriefs with academic researchers, local and cross-site analysis workshops and the final presentation of our national findings by two co-researchers. Our starting approach acknowledged that at an individual level all researchers would begin to analyse soon after collecting data. Each member of the academic research team aimed to capture the development of these ideas among co-researchers in the local site. For instance, after one interview a co-researcher with autism reflected on the different nature of services: how some were essential (housing) and others lower level (football). His concern for our analysis was that people using 'essential' services could demonstrate much more impact in their feedback, while the lower-level services, although they were valued, did not elicit the same powerful responses from service users. This consideration was one that the whole team returned to and developed throughout the analytical and writing process. Ongoing co-researcher observations during the training and in post-interview debriefs were recorded as 'memos' and integrated into the QSR-NVivo analysis, allowing the integration of interview data with emerging ideas from the research (Silverman, 2013).

Analysis workshops with co-researchers were designed as interactive and visual sessions to reveal how co-researchers had interpreted the data they had collected and their ongoing reflections addressing our four hypotheses. During the events the co-researchers generated memos as Post-It notes that were incorporated into the broader analysis by using NVivo memo functions or creating additional codes. The local site sessions were key to gathering people's thoughts about what each service was doing well and what was valued by service users. Local workshops also examined broader contextual issues, often about provision that seemed to be missing. One co-researcher commented:

> "Because there are so many Asian people that live in [local area]. But you go to the day centre and they are not there, even when they've relocated their building to the middle of that community [BME], why is that?" (Co-researcher and carer, North West, excerpt from local analysis workshop)

A national cross-site workshop used a graphic artist to capture the discussions of co-researchers – both how they found the experience of undertaking the research and what they thought the findings should be. Bringing together all the researchers at the local and national events displayed the differences between individual co-researcher perspectives. For instance, we saw that different co-researchers had different attitudes to the potential risks of a micro-enterprise approach. Some co-researchers felt that regulation was crucial to quality and public trust, while others felt that the actual impact of regulation on quality was minimal and the regulatory processes were intrusive. In these sessions, older co-researchers and those with learning disabilities often brought distinctive perspectives and said that they welcomed the opportunity to explore their experiences with such a diverse group. This perhaps suggests that there would be some benefits in combining different 'categories' of co-researchers, where this is appropriate, in future studies, rather than focusing on a certain service user group.

Interview notes, co-researcher memos and transcripts were uploaded to QSR-NVivo 10, a qualitative data analysis software program for coding. This allowed us to organise the large amount of data that had been collected and also to search the data for key words and issues that arose during analysis (Silverman, 2013). The first step of coding involved 'dissecting the text into manageable and meaningful text segments, with the use of a coding framework' (Attride-Stirling, 2001). The coding framework was underpinned by the theoretical interests guiding the research questions and the data was initially coded around the four research hypotheses outlined in Chapter Three (valued, cost-effective, personalised and innovative). These provided a 'start list' of codes and were developed prior to fieldwork (Miles et al, 2014). Phase 2 coding involved the expansion of this initial coding framework using more 'inductive' coding. This involved the development of sub-themes through the extraction of salient, recurring or significant issues within the initial codes (Attride-Stirling, 2001). Appendix 3, 'Developing the innovation theme codes', displays an example of this level of coding and analysis, showing the expansion of the preliminary code for 'Innovation' through a recoding process that separated out the three distinct types of innovation – 'what', 'how' and 'who' – and identified subcodes within them.

To enhance inter-coder reliability, the early stages of coding were undertaken by the academic researchers as a team of coders, working from printed-out transcripts, before being applied to NVivo. The main codes and themes were also discussed with co-researchers at analysis sessions in each location to test their face validity with people who had taken part in the interviews.

In a third phase, axial coding was undertaken, which involved analysing the relationships between codes and developing sub-categories (Fielding, 2008). To do this, the researchers looked for similarities and 'meaningful relationships' (Corbin and Strauss, 1990) between codes. As Fielding (2008) explains, the first stages of coding can be seen as fragmenting the data, while axial coding brings it back together into a 'web of relationships' (Fielding, 2008: 247). Finally, selective coding was used to select cases and quotes to illustrate major themes for use in the written outputs (Fielding, 2008).

ASCOT survey responses were analysed using IBM SPSS v22 to generate descriptive statistics and crosstabs to compare people's SCRQoL on two of the ASCOT domains and their expected SCRQoL in these areas in the absence of service. The data was analysed to identify any particular quality issues (codes within appropriate and plausible ranges). The main analysis was conducted by comparing key outcomes (our dependent variables) by size of provider (our independent variable) and other key background data. The provider's size was coded as a dichotomy (micro and others) as well as the full range of size coding in the initial analysis. The main limitation was our sample size ($N = 95$), which meant that rather large differences in outcomes, by size of provider, would be needed for results to be statistically significant at conventional levels. Value for money was measured by comparing prices (what an individual spends to purchase services from micro, small, medium and large providers in a given area) with ASCOT survey findings and user and carer accounts of the quality of care provided.

As part of the coding process, all data from interviews and ASCOT was assigned 'identification' codes. This anonymised the data, as each respondent had a unique number, differentiated by the locality in which they were based (e.g. all 100 numbers are in Site 1). These numbers are visible in the respondent quotations in this book, for example 123, 201, 333. Further identification codes allowed analytical queries to be run on the basis of respondent characteristics, with individuals often fitting several of these categories, for example older people, people with learning disabilities, carers, geographic location and so on. Coding also allowed the analysis to examine characteristics of the services such as size and type of service. Where we have given more detailed examples of case studies in text boxes we have used anonymised names of people and organisations rather than numbers to enhance readability.

Conclusion

This chapter has provided an overview of our approach to research methods, with a particular focus on the involvement of co-researchers. Although the initial bid for this study, including its methods, was conceived by academic researchers, any reflection on methodology cannot be separated from the involvement of co-researchers. Our commitment to include service users and carers as part of the team at as many stages as possible challenged us to have a more fluid approach to research plans. We revised our methods, modes of analysis and how we might present our findings. An evaluation by colleagues highlighted several benefits of co-researcher involvement. Our learning for future studies has focused on allowing more time to address the training needs of diverse groups of service users, tailoring this individually where appropriate. Our co-productive approach to the research has also suggested the value of making time to have very open conversations with co-researchers, both as groups and individually. These open exchanges often led to new opportunities for the study, helped to bring out richer analytical insights and aligned the thoughts and approaches of academics and co-researchers.

FIVE

What it means to be micro

Chapter Two considered the existing evidence relating to organisational size and performance, and examined the implications when applied to the context of social care. Size was considered as an independent variable whose relationship with organisational performance could be tested through qualitative and quantitative research, even while recognising that sometimes the preferred size of an organisation was driven by management fashion rather than an evidence base. The assumption that size was an observable and measurable variable was the starting point for our research, and remained the underlying premise for testing the four hypotheses about micro–enterprises: that they were likely to produce valued outcomes, and to be more cost–effective, personalised and innovative than larger organisations. The findings chapters that follow this one outline what the research told us about those aspects of organisational performance.

This chapter offers a somewhat different perspective, setting out a range of issues linked to what it means to be micro, and the organisational identities evident within that. Through a discussion of the approach we took to sampling, it highlights the practical dilemmas attendant in identifying and working with organisations whose size was not fixed and stable over the life of the research. The chapter also considers the different governance structures within the organisations that we included in the study, which themselves can be captured as a set of organisational identities as well as legal forms. These included sole traders and partnerships, as well as charities, limited companies and statutory providers. The chapter draws on interview data to look at the motivations people had for setting up particular types of organisation, helping to illuminate the implications of having different organisational types within local care markets. It also uses the data to highlight how size and organisational type was part of the identity of these providers, with the identity of micro, for example, being embraced as a form of distinction both from larger providers in their locality and from social care's institutionalised past.

Finding micro-enterprises

The total number of care sector micro-enterprises in England is not known. Skills for Care data suggests that the numbers are over 6,000 – although its figures are likely to be an underestimate, since they do not include sole traders and those self-employed people who are not eligible for VAT. For our study we aimed to develop a sample of 18 micro-enterprises (6 per locality) in each of the three sites where the research was being undertaken. These micro-enterprises were to be compared with three larger organisations in each area (one small, one medium, one large), making 27 organisations in total. This over-representation of micro-enterprises in the sample reflects the dual aim of the research: to better understand the micro-enterprise sector, as well as to undertake comparative research with small, medium and large care providers. It also reflects the existence of a body of research about attributes of care service providers in which micro-enterprises are not well represented (for example, CQC, 2015). By having a total of 27 organisations in the study and interviewing a staff member, a family carer and three people using services in each organisation, we felt we could generate a large amount of data while keeping the fieldwork at a level that was manageable within a two-year research project.

To identify micro-enterprise in the three localities, we started with the Skills for Care database of care providers (the National Minimum Data Set (NMDS)), which is searchable by locality and size of organisation. Although we could not have access to the full data set, Skills for Care generated lists of providers within the three localities based on the size bandings that we gave them. Organisational size was categorised by the number of staff registered to work in the organisation.

We initially planned to categorise micro, small, medium and large organisations by drawing on the thresholds of the UK Companies Act 2006 (micro, 0–5 FTE; small, 6–50 FTE; medium, 51–250 FTE; large, 251+ FTE). However, the Skills for Care data (2015, p 13) on the size of the sector showed that only 2% of total care providers have over 250 FTE staff. We revised our bandings so that a large company was over 100 FTE staff; companies of this size constitute 6% of the sector (Skills for Care, 2015). Medium-sized companies were classed in our banding as having 51–100 FTE staff (capturing 9% of care companies in England).

The data generated from the NMDS for our three localities is given in Table 5.1.

Table 5.1: Size of care providers by locality

Location	Number of organisations	Size of organisation* breakdown (n and percentage)
Urban local authority in the North West	83	Micro: 1 (1%) Small: 64 (77%) Medium: 13 (16%) Large: 5 (6%)
Two local authorities in the West Midlands with mixed urban and rural profile	399	Micro: 71 (18%) Small: 286 (72%) Medium: 38 (9%) Large: 4 (1%)
Rural county in the East Midlands	597	Micro: 101 (17%) Small: 400 (67%) Medium: 74 (12%) Large: 22 (4%)
All sites	1079	Micro: 173 (16%) Small: 750 (70%) Medium: 125 (11%) Large: 31 (3%)

Note: * Micro: 0–5 FTE; small: 6–50 FTE; medium: 51– 100 FTE; large 101+ FTE.
Source: Adapted from the National Minimum Data Set, Skills for Care.

The data showed a large variation in the number of care providers by locality, although this in part reflects the differential sizes of the localities (for example, a small metropolitan borough versus a larger and more populous county), so we do not make any inferences based on the total numbers in the different areas. However, the very small number of micro-organisations in the North West borough generated doubts in our minds about the effectiveness of the database in capturing micro-enterprises. We knew already that some sole traders and self-employed people would be excluded. However, the figures from the NMDS did not match Skills for Care's own annual estimates of the size of the micro sector. We therefore sought other sources of information about micro-enterprise activity in the three areas. We requested access to local lists of micro-enterprises held by the local authorities or community and voluntary sector organisations. In each of the three localities there was a micro-enterprise coordinator supported by the local authority, usually as a joint appointment with the local authority and Community Catalysts (the national support organisation for micro-enterprises). These coordinators provide start-up advice to care sector micro-enterprises and also convene forums where micro-enterprises can come together for peer support. They shared with us lists and contact details for the local micro-enterprises. The numbers of micro-enterprises on their lists ranged from 30 to 60 per locality – offering a large-enough group of organisations in each area for us to develop a sample of six in each area.

In selecting the micro-enterprise sample from the micro-coordinators' lists – in preference to the Skills for Care database – we were alert to the point made by Mohan et al in the context of their own non-profit sector research: 'what you find out depends on where you look; put another way, listings will undoubtedly reflect the capacities and priorities of those compiling them and the willingness of local organisations to comply with the process of compiling them' (Mohan et al, 2010, p 15). As acknowledged in a previous chapter, working off a list meant that we were able to include only those organisations that operated 'above the radar' and were known to the local authority. The micro-enterprise coordinators had compiled the lists on the basis of people who had approached them for advice and support, or people that they knew about through their own local networks. Using these lists allowed us to generate a sample of micro-enterprises quickly, and to rapidly establish a relationship with the selected micro-enterprise, brokered by the coordinator. We recognise that there are other methodologies through which such organisations can be found independently by the researcher, involving a longer immersion in the local setting, but the time-scales and scope of this project did not allow for this more ethnographic approach. The lists provided by the coordinators were diverse and lengthy enough for us to feel confident in using them to derive a picture of what micro-enterprises can bring to the care sector.

The lists gave an insight into the wide range of different types of care-related micro-enterprises operating in the localities. As well as the organisations that seemed to fit recognisable categories – those providing domiciliary care, day centres and residential settings – there were drama, dance, bread making, pet-based therapies and days out fishing. To reduce these to a sample of six in each area that would be broadly comparable across the three sites, we had to introduce criteria that flattened some of this diversity. Following Wagenaar, we aimed to *'sample for relevant diversity – relevant, that is, in the light of your research question'* (Wagenaar, 2011, p 270, emphasis in original). For us this meant sampling organisations that could help to reflect the diversity of services offered by micro-enterprises, but also illuminate the question of how far they delivered improved outcomes and more innovative, personalised and cost-effective services than larger providers did. To an extent, therefore, we had to choose services that had a broadly comparable equivalent in a large provider. We started by clustering the micro-enterprises under headings that are well-established in the social care sector: residential care; personal care in the home (that is, washing and dressing type activities regulated by the CQC); and day activities outside the home. However, it became clear that these activities – all defined by the spatial context in which they take place – were inadequate in their coverage of the support offered by many of the micro-enterprises. We therefore separated the 'day activities' category into scheduled group activities and one-to-one support for individuals. This latter category might cover 'home help' type activities, but also taking people out for the day. An example of this type of support is given in an interview with a family carer, talking about someone from a micro-enterprise who supports her mum.

> "She'll literally do anything you ask of her. And she's taking mum out now, she bought the wheelchair that she'd used for somebody else ... She's taken mum out, you know, just to pop down the shops to get a few bits if mum wants anything and just to get out the place ... If there's nothing to be done and she can't take mum out, she'll find something and she involves mum." (Carer 103, Micro one-to-one support)

Having established four categories of service type (domiciliary, residential, group day activities and one-to-one support), we developed additional purposive sampling criteria drawn from aspects of diversity within the social care sector and highlighted by the literature reviews that preceded the fieldwork. These sampling criteria are shown in Box 5.1

Box 5.1: Sampling criteria for micro-enterprises
- Supporting older people and/or people with learning disabilities
- Type of service (domiciliary care; day activities; residential care; one-to-one support)
- 'Mainstream' services and those targeted at diverse user groups (for example, BME; lesbian, gay, bisexual and transgender (LGBT)
- CQC-registered and non-registered
- Purchased by local authority; personal budget holder; self-funder
- Number of years of operating
- Number of staff
- Governance type (sole trader, limited company, charity and so on)
- User led and non user led

In the each of the three sites, we worked with the local micro-enterprise coordinators to identify a sample of 6 micro-enterprises that best fitted our sampling frame, so that across the 18 we got a balance across these criteria as far as this was possible. There were very few residential micro-enterprises on the coordinators' lists, for example, so only one residential micro was included in the research. We also needed to work with organisations that had at least three or four regular users who had used the service for a minimum of several months, to enable them to comment on its quality. The micro-enterprise coordinators flagged up to us that some of the more innovative-sounding micro-enterprises were very new or lacked that established base of users. This limitation meant that some innovative-sounding micro-enterprises – a fishing group for men with dementia; an LGBT-oriented social group – could not be used as case studies.

There were some other barriers to operationalising the sampling frame. We aimed to select organisations that offered support to older people and to adults with learning disabilities. However, micro-enterprises did not always tailor their offer to particular 'client groups', and therefore to speak to the people using its services we had to go outside the older people and learning disability categories and include a small number of people with other impairments, such as autism. Some micro-enterprises operated inside local authority premises, blurring the lines between sectors. We struggled to find organisations that provided LGBT-oriented support, and were able to include only three organisations that had a BME focus.

Once we had identified micro-enterprises on the list that met our sampling criteria, then the coordinators provided contact details and allowed us to use their names when approaching the organisations. Having the credentials of this contact helped us to convince the micro-enterprises to work with us. Nonetheless, we sometimes had to go back to the lists to find replacements because the organisations on the list were either too small or too big to be appropriate for the evaluation: one micro-enterprise withdrew from the project at a late stage, meaning that we ended up with 17 rather than 18 organisations.

Finding small, medium and large providers

So much research into the social care sector highlights the limitations of the services provided (often due to lack of money as much as anything else) that we were unsure whether small, medium and large providers would agree to the level of scrutiny necessitated by taking part in a research study. In approaching them we did not have the 'in' that was given to us by the micro-coordinator. Since the project had 'micro-enterprise' in its title, it was clear that we were interested in these larger organisations only for comparative purposes. Given the anticipated difficulties of recruiting these organisations, we delayed these interviews until after we had completed the fieldwork with the micro-enterprises, by which time we had developed local contacts who helped us to identify potential contributors. For example, local authority commissioners and local charities shared with us the e-mail addresses of small, medium and large care providers and an assurance that we could use their name within the e-mail to help encourage a positive response.

We aimed for three small, three medium and three large organisations (one of each size in each site). The sample that emerged had four small, four medium and two large organisations. Some of these were stand-alone organisations, while others were franchises of large charities or companies. This is a further limitation of working with size as a variable, as discussed in Chapter Two. Organisations are not discrete and firmly bounded institutions waiting to be researched. They are clusters of people and functions, and where to draw the boundaries of the organisation is a necessary part of the research process. We recognised that the number of staff employed by an organisation could be measured at the service unit (such as a care home or a day centre), or across a locality, nationally or internationally. Where small local organisations belong to larger groups it can be difficult to classify them. Some large chains involve hands-on control from the board of directors, others are mergers that continue on a more federated basis. As Sheaff et al note, 'Mergers that simply federate organisations which otherwise retain separate core working activities and physical resources are likely to make little practical difference to the productivity or efficiency of their constituent organisations' (Sheaff, 2004). Franchises similarly can operate with a large degree of freedom from their parent organisations. Buckingham (2012) notes that, 'Federal organisations, where a local TSO (Third Sector Organisation) was affiliated to a larger national organisation … were able to draw on the resources of the national organisations, but otherwise exhibited attributes more akin to the "grassroots' providers".'

Three of the organisations that we selected for inclusion in the project were part of large national organisations (one charity, one social enterprise and one for-profit provider). We had to decide whether to classify these organisations on the basis of the size of the office in the locality or by the size of the national organisation. In our staff interviews, all of them reported high degrees of independence from their parent organisation. The validity of considering the local office as the unit of analysis is confirmed in the work of Considine, who in his comparative work on public and private providers of public services points to 'local offices as the primary locus for differences in staff and client behaviour' (Considine, 2000, p 279). We decided therefore to classify organisations by the size in the locality rather than according to their national profile. In making this choice we of course recognise that such a perspective is imperfect: a stand-alone day service is not directly comparable with one that operates under the banner of a national charity. However, given that our focus was on the quality of support provided to people within that locality, we felt that the local size of the organisation was the key unit of analysis. We do, though, return to issues of franchises and national chains later in the book.

Table 5.2 shows the service types that were included in the sample by organisational size. The balance between types of service reflects that of the micro-enterprise lists we were given by the coordinators, in which residential and domiciliary care were relatively under-represented, as compared to day activities and one-to-one support. It also reflects the extent to which we were able to recruit different types and sizes of provider to take part in the research. For example, we found it particularly difficult to recruit large domiciliary care agencies as participants in the project. In one locality the high turnover of senior staff in such an agency meant that contacts had to be re-established several times during the fieldwork phase of the project, leading us eventually to give up and contact another provider.

Table 5.2: The sample of organisations, by size and service type

	Domiciliary	Residential	Group day activities	One-to-one support	Total
Micro	3	1	8	5	17
Small	3	0	1	0	4
Medium	0	1	2	1	4
Large	1	0	1	0	2
Total	7	2	12	6	27

Note: * Micro: 0–5 FTE; small: 6–50 FTE; medium: 51–100 FTE; large 101+ FTE.
Size categories are adapted from the UK C Companies Act 2006.

Organisational types

As well as varying by their size and the types of service provided, the organisations we selected differed in their legal structure and governance arrangements. Table 5.3 shows the range of different types of organisation that took part in the research.

Table 5.3: The sample of organisations, by size and legal form

	Local authority	Charity	CIC	Sole trader/ partnership	Limited company	Total
Micro	0	2	1	9	5	17
Small	0	1	0	0	3	4
Medium	1	3	0	0	0	4
Large	1	0	0	0	1	2
Total	2	6	1	9	9	27

Note: * Micro: 0–5 FTE; small: 6–50 FTE; medium: 51– 100 FTE; large 101+ FTE.
Size categories are adapted from the UK C Companies Act 2006.

As set out in Chapters Two and Three, successive governments since the Thatcher era have pushed increasing numbers of social care services out of public ownership into the for-profit and not-for-profit sectors. The mix of sectors in our sample is broadly typical of patterns in adult social care services: in England two-thirds of social care staff are employed by the private sector, with one fifth employed by the third sector and only one tenth employed in the statutory sector (Skills for Care, 2015).

Like organisational size and performance, the relationship between legal form and performance has been of interest for public management scholars, although findings have been inconclusive (Hill and Lynn, 2005). There are some studies – such as Considine (2000) – that compare public, non-profit and for-profit providers of the same service (employment assistance), but even in those studies it is issues relating to results-based funding rather than formal governance structures that explain sectoral differences.

The different legal forms in our sample highlight the need to separate out the aggregate headings of private sector or third sector provider that have been used in much public management literature. Sole traders and limited companies are bundled together in such arrangements (in practice probably because sole traders are not included at all), whereas in our research we were able to disaggregate them into distinct categories. Existing research on the self-employed affirms the difference between the attitudes and behaviours of these individuals and larger firms (Dellot, 2015; Mallett and Wapshott, 2015). While literature on organisational identity has highlighted the extent to which it can be separated out from personal identity (Hatch and Schultz, 1997), this is less the case with very small organisations and sole traders, where self-identity can become tied up with being an 'entrepreneur' (Watson, 2009). Mallett and Wapshott (2015, p 262) refer to the constant struggle and 'inevitable ups and downs that self-employment entails', and this can require considerable commitment and attachment leading to a higher level of self-identification with the business.

Table 5.4 shows the organisational type by the service provided, which highlights that local authorities and charities mainly provide group day services rather than other kinds of services. Limited companies predominantly provide domiciliary care and sole traders are split between providing group day services and one-to-one support. Of the service types, the one that is most split between organisational types is group day activities.

Table 5.4: The sample of organisations, by service type and legal form

	Local authority	Charity	CIC	Sole trader/ partnership	Limited company	Total
Domiciliary	0	0	0	0	7	7
Group day activities	2	4	1	4	1	12
Residential	0	1	0	1	0	2
One-to-one support	0	1	0	4	1	6
Total	2	6	1	9	9	27

Looking at the different governance types in turn can help to generate insights into the distinctive features of operating within those sectors, and also the different ways in which organisations relate to their identity.

Local authority

Direct provision of care and support services by local authorities is increasingly rare. The two local authority providers that we included were both day centres – one for older people and the other for people with learning disabilities. In the interviews with people running these services there was a language of managed decline in what they offer now, compared to the past. However, this was not necessarily seen by managers as problematic, as it could stimulate new ways of working:

> "If we have a cut of, I don't know, £30,000 from the budget, we say OK, how can we work without that to enable services to be a little bit more preventative, do you know what I mean? So rather than providing care, we provide an access – we become a hub I suppose ... we've sort of pressed on with the transition of enabling people who use the services to become involved. So I suppose what we've done is we've developed the sort of more exciting user-led side of the service, which in a way has by coincidence compensated for the fact that we've had less money." (Staff 111, Medium day service)

In another locality, the coming together of different types of users in one large day centre as several smaller ones closed was felt by the manager to not only reduce costs but also overcome the barriers that might exist, for example between older people and young people with learning disabilities.

On the whole we did not identify relevant differences between the three localities in the research, finding size of organisation a more powerful explanatory variable than place. However, there was a discernible difference between the local authorities in the three localities in terms of their attitudes to the outsourcing of services, which is important to bring out. In one of the three localities, there had been a determined effort to retain or bring back 'in-house' services. In contrast, the ownership of care services did not seem to be as politically salient in the other two localities, both of which had outsourced the vast bulk of social care.

The Labour Party was the majority or biggest party in all of the local authorities in the study, so this cannot simply be explained as a party-political difference. As has been argued elsewhere, personalisation exposes tensions between different kinds of progressive politics: the pro-public sector instincts of parts of the political Left, and the pro-community self-help politics of other parts (Needham, 2011). This Old Left vs New Left politics invokes different bogeymen: advocates of in-house provision can see micro-enterprises as examples of grassroots neoliberalism in which people using and providing services are forced to operate as exemplars of the 'entrepreneurial self' (Kelly, 2006; see also Gordon, 1991; Burchell, 1996; Scourfield, 2007). For the micro-providers and disability campaigners promoting personalisation more broadly, in-house provision can be seen as protectionism and paternalism that diminishes the citizenship of people with disabilities (Duffy, 2014).

Two of the micro-enterprises in our study had been set up by people at the same time as they were working for local authority care services. Here there was a fascinating difference of attitude between the two local authorities where the micro-enterprises were based. One of the local authorities was explicitly encouraging staff to set up spin-offs, as a way of skilling up staff to mitigate the risks associated with further workforce shrinkage. The two people running the micro-enterprise continued to work full time at a local authority day centre and ran the micro-enterprise in their evenings and at weekends (providing a sitting service and transport). Some of their referrals came from the day centre attendees and staff, and the day centre manager was happy for this to continue, so long as they did not take calls for their business during work hours and there was no direct competition between the service they were offering and that provided by the day centre:

> "There was some debate about whether we would be allowed to do it from the corporate side but we quickly established that we weren't in direct competition to what we were doing in the day. We weren't providing day care, we weren't doing personal care ..." (Staff 109, Micro one-to-one support)

In the other local authority, a staff member who had set up a micro-enterprise was disciplined by senior managers and (in her perception) every effort was made to discourage her from continuing with it: "I got various people's support in the council to get the CQC registration, and then someone senior found out and I was hauled up. We aren't allowed to be on the commissioners' list of preferred providers. And that's been set for five years." (Staff 6a, Micro day service) A colleague in her micro-enterprise reflected: "It has been difficult to promote ourselves because of [the colleague's] role in the council. We weren't allowed to get letters through to day centre people because ... it looked like she was drumming up business for herself." (Staff 6b, Micro day service) As our research was starting the staff member was taking early retirement from the local authority to enable her to concentrate on building up the micro-enterprise.

Some of the difference between the two local authorities is likely to reflect the types of service on offer. In the first case, there was no direct competition between the day centre and the evenings/weekend support that the micro was offering. In the second case, the micro offered a range of different services, including support during the day, which could potentially lead to reduced demand for the day centre. However, there also seemed to be a cultural difference between the two councils' attitudes to spin-outs and staff enterprise and the ethical boundaries attendant within this. Prior research on public service mutuals has referred to the tensions between local authorities and staff trying to spin out their service, with senior management 'buy-in' being crucial to the success or failure of the new enterprise (Hazenberg and Hall, 2014, p 15). In some cases, public sector bodies have resisted spin-outs, often leading to their failure to set started. In other cases public sector bodies have explicitly encouraged staff to spin out. Indeed, Hall et al (2012b) found that some NHS staff were 'pushed' into spinning out their service when threatened with the service being closed or put out to tender.

Sole traders and partnerships

For local authority services, much of the discussion related to why and how the local authorities were reducing their involvement in care services. No one we interviewed from a statutory service was involved in setting up a new in-house service. For the people involved in other types of organisation, we were able to discuss with them the reasons for choosing that particular organisational type. Those who were registered as sole traders or in partnerships were characterised by the degree of control that they had and wanted to retain over their enterprises. Almost all of them had left larger organisations to set up on their own, and these interviewees talked about their businesses very much in terms of individual ownership: "it had been my baby project. I'd set it all up" (Staff 14, Micro day support). The literature indicates that making the move from being employed to self-employed is underpinned by a search for flexibility and individualisation (Fenwick, 2002), and this is evident here. Fenwick (2002) refers to how the move to self-employment can come from a gradual realisation that past jobs were stifling opportunities to exercise creative authority or take initiative.

Interviewees articulated a strong sense of ownership and control over the service, which in some cases led to a reluctance to take on more staff, as one partner reflected:

> "You have got to know that your staff are doing the job as if they were one of us. That can be a barrier to expanding.

When it's us we know what we are delivering." (Staff 104,
Micro one-to-one support)

The sole traders had to manage the trade-offs between their own
availability and reluctance to turn people away:

> "You know, I've worked really hard. I'm getting the work
> and now I've got to give it away. But as [my husband] says,
> I'm only giving it away 'cause I've got other work ... So we
> made a list of the other day, who I've got; who will I give
> away? You know, who will I let somebody else do? But I
> went down the list and I says, 'None of them. Not giving
> them away.' I want them. So I've spread out to weekends
> now." (Staff 101, Micro one-to one support).

Two motivations seemed to be bundled up in this aspiration not to
'give people away'. First, there was the desire to retain business, since
it was this individual's only source of income. Second, there was an
attachment to the people, which meant that she wanted to continue
to offer them support: "Me gentleman I do now, he's all right to let
somebody cover. But there's some that I wouldn't. You know. You get
attached." (Staff 101, Micro one-to-one support).

Limited companies

Several of the people we spoke to had set up as limited companies.
This included micro, small, medium and large examples. For some of
the micro-enterprises, the decision to go down the limited company
route was to retain control of the organisation:

> "If I became a charitable status then I would lose control of
> my business, if I was to sit on the management committee
> then that would mean I wouldn't be able to work for my
> business or vice versa." (Staff 303, Micro day service)

One interviewee from a limited company talked about charitable status
as a back-up if the business approach failed:

> "We've had the year's books back from the accountant
> who said obviously you're running at a loss and you need
> to decide, well, it's not really about that. So we'll probably
> see how it goes this year and see whether it can maintain

itself and then if not we'll have to look at perhaps going down the charity route. Because you can't get, because we're classed as a business we can't get any funding." (Staff 302, Micro day service)

This quote highlights the flexibility of organisational types – people had often opted pragmatically for a particular governance structure when they started out, perhaps because money was more readily available for that type of organisation – but were willing to shift if circumstances made a different organisational type more likely to survive.

This sense of organisational identities as flexible and overlapping rather than fixed and discrete was brought out in an interview we did with a home care provider operating at the boundary of small and medium, and part of a large national franchise of home care providers. What was interesting in the interview was the way in which the interviewee tracked between articulation of the organisation as a family firm and as a franchise of a national brand. In the early part of the interview the respondent said:

"It's very much like an old–fashioned family business where it doesn't matter how big we get in X number of years' time. It will never be different because we will always take the time to visit all of our clients and see them on a regular basis and to stay in touch with all the care givers on a regular basis." (Staff 112, Small domiciliary care)

And later in the interview:

Respondent: [Our company] is rated number one in terms of compliance for the whole of the UK across all of the national care companies which is for elderly people receiving domiciliary care ...

Interviewer: So is your feeling if I went to interview somebody at [another franchise of the same company] in the neighbouring set of postcodes, we'd have a similar kind of conversation?

Respondent: I would have thought so, yes ... I would hope so. (Staff 112, Small domiciliary care)

This point highlights the need to acknowledge the multiple and interlocking organisational identities through which people explain and give value to what they do. As this chapter shows, organisational forms and identities are not fixed, affirming the importance of recognising unstable organisational boundaries that was discussed in Chapter Two. Young (2001) refers to different types of for-profit organisations, based on their degree of social responsibility. This includes 'corporate philanthropists', where philanthropic activities contribute towards organisational productivity, or a 'social purpose organisation', which, while considered a private organisation, devotes itself to achieving some social good. These organisational forms can also fall under the (often vague) category of 'social enterprise' (discussed further below) and further indicate the way in which organisations can possess multiple, overlapping identities.

Social enterprise

Only one of the micro-enterprise case studies had taken an organisational form that is explicitly a social enterprise. It was set up as a CIC, which, through an 'asset lock' and 'community interest statement', serves to benefit the community rather than private shareholders (HM Government, 2015). However, the blurred boundaries of what it means to be a social enterprise are well known (for example, Teasdale, 2011), as discussed above.

Some other organisations, while not CICs, also took an explicit 'social enterprise' route in part of their activity, as the quote from a staff member in a local authority day service indicates:

> "We run probably 10 community cafes now which are all not-for-profit-based social enterprises and all the money and the proceeds for that go back into the service. They allow people to have real-life working opportunities ... So they help with the numeracy and literacy, customer skills – so it ticks a lot of boxes for somebody who is looking into employment." (Staff 207, Large day service)

Many of the micro-enterprises expressed a strong social mission, identifying with the characteristics of a social enterprise while not explicitly being one. This centred on the desire to combine profit making with an ethos of care.

> "I run a business and I want to make a profit, but in our hearts we know what we want to give and I say to each member of staff – it sounds a bit hard, but – 'If you don't

give me the quality of work that my own son would be happy with …'." (Staff 103, Micro domiciliary care)

We encountered this tension – balancing a care ethos with sufficient income to keep going – in many of the interviews, and return to it later in the book.

Charities

Six of the case study organisations were set up as not-for-profit charities. These ranged in size from micro to medium. Charities tend to have a much more distinct organisational brand and identity than some of the other organisational forms discussed above. Most charities, including those in our study, tend to be heavily reliant on donations and volunteers, which they are able to achieve through a strong pro-social image and reputation focused on compassion, idealism and a focus on beneficiaries (Bennett and Gabriel, 2003). This was evident in our case study charities, who sometimes articulated this as an ethic of care:

> "Well I think [we] started 30 years ago because parents and a psychologist said people have no choice and people have no activities, you know, … that during the day, you know, there's no choice for people with learning disabilities. And that's always been the underpinning priority for the charity." (Staff 205, Micro day service)

Other interviewees from charities were more pragmatic in their motivation for going down the charitable route, feeling that the charity 'brand' helped in getting access to funding and clients:

> "In some respects, I wish I'd set this up as a private enterprise and sold it as a franchise … I think the reason I set it up as a charity is because I knew that older people would use the service if it was a charity and, at the time I set it up, there was quite a lot of funding that was available, I got a social enterprise grant from the county council … and I knew if we would get the county council logo on the back of it, that would be it." (Staff 304, Micro day service)

Operating as a charity shaped the ways in which people ran and charged for the service, which at times could be detrimental:

"I think we should have put the prices up more but it was alien to the charity to actually charge people to do things and although your head says, you think oh, you know, people may struggle and we're in hugely challenged times and people's budgets are being reviewed very robustly by the council. And in some cases rightly, you know. So I think we will start to put an annual increase in just to keep abreast of inflation because we're just about covering our costs on it." (Staff 205, Micro day service)

There was here, then, the same tension as expressed by other organisational types between the mission of the organisation – to help people whose own care budgets were being reduced – and the need to ensure that the organisation was financially sustainable.

User-led organisations

As discussed in Chapter Three, a key thrust of recent social care sector reforms has been to move towards a more co-productive approach in which people who use services and are family carers are more involved in the design and delivery of support. In Chapter Eight this will be discussed as part of the innovative aspects of micro-enterprise, as an example of *who* innovation. Here, in relation to legal form, it is noteworthy that we did find some micro-enterprises that were set up by people who used services or that had a strong involvement of people with disabilities in their governance structures. Both of these characteristics were particularly a feature of day services for people with learning disabilities. We did not encounter any organisations for older people that were user led or involved older people in their governance structures. This may be a feature of our sample, which did not include any information, advocacy or advice services, where there may be more scope for older people to be involved in organisational management (SCIE, 2012; NDTI, 2013). It may also be an issue of classification and listing, reprising the point made by Mohan et al (2010, p 15). above, about how the results you get are shaped by where you look. We recruited the micro-enterprise organisations from lists held by micro-enterprise coordinators, whose role included small business support. If we had instead approached the teams within adult social care services that work on community inclusion, we might have had more user-led organisations brought to our attention.

Conclusion

In this chapter we have considered how to work with size as a variable for research. The discussion affirmed the difficulties of operationalising size, and the need to work with context-specific rather than generalised size categories. This insight shaped which organisations were invited to take part in the research. The chapter has also considered the different organisational forms that were found among the micro-enterprises, covering sole traders and partnerships, charities, social enterprises and limited companies. It has highlighted the ways in which people running these organisations articulated the identities that accompanied them, and why they had selected particular organisational forms. The discomfort that many of these organisations felt about making a profit from care services has been set alongside the need to ensure financial sustainability. This issue of making micro-enterprises financially stable is returned to in Chapter Ten when we consider the likelihood that such organisations can play a key role in future social care provision.

SIX

Micro-enterprises: better outcomes at a lower cost

The previous chapters have considered how and why to study size, the participative approach taken in the research study and the organisational identities at work among our case study micro-enterprises. The next three chapters present the findings from the research, focused on the four hypotheses. The issue of whether micro-enterprises achieve better outcomes and value for money than larger providers is considered in this chapter. The next chapter looks at the process of care and whether micro-enterprises are more personalised in the support they provide than larger care providers. Chapter Eight considers whether or not they are more innovative. These chapters draw primarily on different dominant data sources. This chapter utilises two main data sources: the quantitative outcomes data gathered from the ASCOT survey and the pricing data given to us by the organisations – although qualitative interview data is also brought in so as to better understand these quantitative findings. In the next chapter, the personalisation section draws predominantly on interview data from people using services and family carers. The innovation chapter draws most heavily on the staff interviews that we did for the project. Here we begin by setting out the findings about outcomes of care, and then go on to compare outcomes with pricing data to establish how far micro-enterprises offer value for money as compared to larger providers.

Care outcomes

In Chapter Two we set out six ways of measuring performance, covering output quality and quantity, efficiency, value for money, outcomes and consumer satisfaction. For several years now, measurement of the performance of public services has focused on the outcomes that they deliver over other measures of performance (Commission for Social Care Inspection, 2006; DH, 2006; Wanless, 2006). Outcomes are presented as a move away from a naïve focus on outputs (number of care visits a day, number of operations performed), which can hide poor-quality service. Outcomes are more sophisticated: in relation to social care they are 'the valued consequences of social care support for service users and other people', and include quality of life and well-being (Caiels et al, 2010, p 1). As Caiels et al point out: 'measuring wellbeing outcomes, rather than units of service *output* (e.g. the numbers of care home placements), gives us a much better indication of *value*' (2010, p 1). Outcome approaches tend to draw on subjective measures more heavily than do other measures of performance, folding consumer satisfaction in as one way of measuring outcomes.

Outcomes are, however, much more elusive than output or process measures: they are compromised by attribution problems and the absence of counterfactuals (Talbot, 2010). Public policy academics have used terms such as 'outcome theology' and 'fool's gold' to convey this sense that an outcome orientation in performance measurement relies on faith and wishful thinking as much as on hard metrics (Bovaird, 2012; Tunstill and Blewitt, 2013). Bovaird (2012, pp 4–5) draws on the work of Dahler-Larsen (2005), cautioning:

> many 'outcome measures' are chosen by public agencies not because they really correspond to the quality of life improvements which the agency seeks but because they are easy to measure, fashionable, or sympathetically regarded by the controlling political group (or, we would add, in some cases because they are easy to game in performance management or evaluation).

Within a social care setting, outcome measures have tended to focus on quality of life as indicated by whether or not people feel that they have choice and control, and whether or not they can access employment, see friends and have a home life that they are satisfied with. These are inevitably subjective. The nature of social care – its concern with personal care and with how people spend their time – gives primacy to subjective perceptions to a greater degree than in other services such as health, where objective assessments of performance (such as clinical outcomes) carry greater weight. People using social care services are – in formal policy pronouncements at least – recognised to be 'experts on their own lives', which carries over into an assumption that they also know best about whether or not services are performing well (Poll, 2007). For this reason, surveys of people using services have been a commonly used tool to assess outcomes.

As discussed in Chapter Four, we used ASCOT to assess people's SCRQoL. Developed by the University of Kent, ASCOT is one of the best-known and most widely used outcomes measure within social care. It addresses the attribution issue by explicitly asking people about whether or not their care provider helps them to achieve particular outcomes, and whether they would achieve less of a particular outcome if the service was no longer there. Of course there are problems with this approach to outcome measurement, as the research team from Kent acknowledge, such as the absence of a control group against which to test service-related outcomes. However they also highlight the practical, ethical and financial barriers to more robust approaches, such as having a control group that does not have access to the service (Caiels et al, 2010, p 9). A further advantage of ASCOT is now that it is so widely used within social care evaluation (including in the biennial national DH social care survey), which enhances comparability of services and allows findings to be benchmarked against other studies.

However, ASCOT, like many outcome tools, does not gather information about how the outcomes are achieved. As Bovaird points out: 'While providing a useful "summative" evaluation of social care interventions , this approach is "black box" in nature – it provides no understanding of *how* social care (or any other pathway to outcomes) actually produces its effects and therefore gives no guidance on how social care initiatives might be redesigned to improve outcomes' (Bovaird, 2013, p 5). The process of care is hidden. However, for many people receiving care and support: 'quality resides largely in process – that is, the way in which patients are treated' (Day and Klein, 1987, p 386, cited in Lewis and West, 2014, p 4). That is, care is an end in itself rather than a means to achieve another outcome (Mol, 2008; Barnes et al, 2015).

In order to understand the contribution of micro-enterprises, it was important for us to look into this black box. For this reason we combined ASCOT with qualitative interviews in the research. The interviews allowed us to consider the process of care and the ways in which different sizes of provider engaged with the people they were supporting. Several of the people whom we interviewed used more than one care provider, and this further weakened the capacity of ASCOT to help us draw a clear line between the service offered and the outcome achieved. Chapters Seven and Eight in particular focus on these 'black box' aspects of process in relation to care. Here we focus more directly on the outcome data.

Valued outcomes

We investigated the capacity for micro-enterprises to help people to achieve valued outcomes in two ways. The first was to ask people, using ASCOT, whether they felt that using the service gave them more choice and control and more opportunity to spend time doing what they enjoyed than would be the case without the service. Second, in the qualitative analysis, we looked at the extent to which people talked about being able to achieve a valued outcome.

Findings taken from the ASCOT questionnaire show associations between outcomes data and the size of the provider (Table 6.1). The first set of questions related to the extent to which the provider helped people using the service to do more of the things they valued and enjoyed with their time. People were asked to score whether they could do this always, sometimes, rarely or never, and then whether that score would change if they no longer had the support of their care provider.

Table 6.1: Outcomes data for micro-enterprises and other providers compared to national Adult Social Care survey data (%)

Outcome	Micro (n=58)	Others (n=37)	All (n=95)	ASC survey 2013–14
Do you do things you enjoy and value with your time?				
Able to spend as much time as wanted doing things valued or enjoyed	50	22	39	33
Able to do enough of the things valued or enjoyed	33	46	38	33
Do some things valued or enjoyed but not enough	17	30	22	26
Don't do anything valued or enjoyed	–	3	1	7
* Chi-sq(3) = 8.9, p<0.05				
Do the support and services from <provider> affect how you spend your time?				
No	16	7	11	43
Yes	93	84	89	57
Fisher's exact test, p = 0.18 (2-sided)				
Do you feel you have control over your daily life?				
As much control as I want	41	31	37	32
Some control (not enough)	21	25	22	19
Adequate control	38	39	38	44
No control	–	6	2	5
Chi-sq(3) = 4.1, p = 0.25				

Outcome	Micro (n=58)	Others (n=37)	All (n=95)	ASC survey 2013–14
Do the support and services from <provider> affect how much control you have over your daily life?				
No	34	28	32	13
Yes	66	72	68	87
Fisher's exact test, p = 0.65 (2-sided)				

Note: '-' means no cases observed.

Findings from the 95 people who completed ASCOT indicated that those receiving support from a micro-enterprise did tend to be able to do more of the things they valued and enjoyed with their time, and to a significantly greater degree than those receiving care from larger services. These respondents also reported an ability to spend time doing such activities to a greater degree than the average response from the national Adult Social Care Survey 2013–14, run by the DH, which also used ASCOT: 50% of those receiving care from a micro-enterprise in our study were able to spend their time as they wanted, compared with 22% receiving care from larger providers in our study and 33% on average in the national survey (Health and Social Care Information Centre, 2014, p 5).

In terms of the second set of questions (which aimed to surface whether people had more choice and control as a result of receiving services from a given provider) the findings were less conclusive. The data showed that there were some signs that people using micro-enterprises had greater control over their lives than did people using larger services – and that the care provider was making a difference to how much control they felt they had. The answers provided for the micro-providers in our study (41% having as much control as they would like) were above those for the larger providers (31%) and above the national average of 33% (Health and Social Care Information Centre, 2014, p 4). However, these variations between providers are not large enough to have confidence in any statistical differences.

We drew on the qualitative interview data to further assess whether or not people talked about a tangible improvement or benefit from using the service, which could be classified as an improved outcome (or, conversely, a worsened outcome due to a problem with the service). In relation to social isolation, for example, this interviewee highlighted the benefits received from attending a weekly football session in a micro–enterprise led by another person with learning disabilities:

> "I go there to interact and exercise. You know it's better than just sat on my computer all day. If I can go out and interact with people, you know, it's going to help me to go out in the future. Like I say if I get a job or I go back to college again … It gets a bit boring when you're just sat at home and there's no one to speak to. You get a bit, don't know, it just it's a bit sad isn't it?" (Person with learning disabilities 203, Micro day service)

Box 6.1 gives another example of a person achieving a valued outcome through support offered by a micro–enterprise. However, in most of the interviews there was no real articulation of a particular outcome separate from the process by which the care was delivered.

Box: 6.1 A valued outcome

Your Support is a micro-enterprise that was set up by an autism specialist and provides employment experience for people with different educational needs. The organisation employs one of the people who also uses the service, taking what it describes as a co-productive approach. The micro-enterprise states its aims as being to empower people with autism and make connections to similar networks in the region. It offers one-to-one sessions that vary from person to person. Activities can include: goal setting and working toward employment; physical activities and days out; and social and peer group activities.

An interviewee who uses this service described to us how he gets to choose the activities he enjoys most and how the service has supported him to achieve the personal goal of having more friends:

> "It's more choice in what you want to do. Whereas before I've not always had that, you know. I have a weekly planner what I want to do…. I mean the goals are getting more friends, things like that … you know just being happier really. I just wanted to be settled and I have got more friends now." (Person with learning disabilities 224, Micro day service)

In explaining the differences between the people who articulated a distinctive outcome that they wanted from the care service and those who focused more on the care as an end in itself, there were differences by type of service user and location of care: it was older people in the home, in particular, who struggled to articulate an outcome beyond getting good-quality care. In the interviews with younger people and their family carers there was more likely to be discussion of an end result (such as making new friends, building confidence, getting fit, finding a job) that was distinguishable from the support that made it happen. This was also more the case with the older people who attended a day activity, some of whom, for example, placed value on getting to know people or gained personal satisfaction from engaging in memory workshops or art classes.

For people who were able to identify an outcome, there was no clear pattern about whether these outcomes were more likely to be achieved by using micro-enterprises or by the larger organisations. There were examples of valued outcomes being achieved across all the different-sized organisations. However, this was often contingent on there being a particular individual who had taken the time to support people towards a mutually identified goal, as this example highlights:

> "[H]is support worker realised that [the person using the service] likes – he's quite big on the cleaning side of it. He started volunteering to clean people's cars. He's now got his own cul-de-sac of people that he spends his day cleaning their cars, he does a bit of gardening, he puts the bins out … And the community have all chipped in and bought him some gear to do it and we're now hoping that he's going to become self-employed." (Staff 207, Large day service)

This quote, which begins with the support worker as the catalyst, reinforces the importance of secure and consistent interpersonal relationships to achieving good outcomes, a theme that is discussed in more detail in the next chapter. This can sometimes be achieved by larger providers, as it is in the example above, or by a micro-enterprise, as in this next interview extract, in which the interviewee discusses the support he received following the death of his father. He compares the response of the micro-enterprise that provides his accommodation (the landlord) with the input he received from the local authority learning disability support service.

> "[H]e [the landlord] could say 'well it's not my problem, you're on your own', but he's actually sticking his neck out and helping me out, whereas [the local authority] team, I feel as though they have abandoned me, just keeping on the

books to make them look good." (Person with a learning disability 216, Micro accommodation service)

The importance of being outcomes focused was something that a lot of the staff interviewees were well aware of. However, not all of the organisations wanted to be too rigidly focused on the achievement of externally established outcomes. As the organiser of one day service put it:

> "We'll say to people 'what would you like to do', so we've had bake-offs, Italian days, cowboy days ... sometimes there is a criticism that these are, you know, we're supposed to be developing life skills and independent living ... and we say 'well actually we don't want to spend the whole of our days bettering and improving ourselves, we want to have a bit of fun, we want to do things we enjoy ... you know, it doesn't all have to be let's learn to write and how to travel on a bus." (Staff 215, Micro day service)

There are, then, some limitations in assessing care in relation to externally determined outcomes: not all people using services have a recognised goal they can articulate beyond 'good care' and not all people want to accept a potentially narrow view of what constitutes an outcome.

Outcomes for carers

As well as outcomes for the people directly in receipt of support, family carers talked about the benefits gained from having a trusted care provider in their home. These outcomes can perhaps best be captured as improvements in well-being for the carer – all the examples below illustrate ways in which people felt supported and cheered by the presence of the care provider. One spouse carer talked about the micro-enterprise that came in to support her husband with dementia:

> "Well it's just lovely for me to sit down for half an hour. I write letters to other carers. I've got five ladies I write to. And it's just my time and while I'm sitting here they're tidying the kitchen up and it's just wonderful." (Carer 102, Micro domiciliary care)

She then talked about how different the experience was with the previous care provider, a large domiciliary care agency, arranged by social services:

> "The people I were having from social services weren't very satisfactory. In fact they weren't very satisfactory at all.... I have cried when they've gone sometimes, because I felt so, you know, this isn't what our last life, our last hours on this earth or days should be you know ... [When the micro-enterprise came in] I thought it was fantastic. The hour they sort of treated us like we were special and we felt better about it. We didn't feel a pest and in the way at all, because they didn't make you feel as though, you know, you feel it's above them looking after old people." (Carer 102, Micro domiciliary care)

According to another family carer of a person supported by a micro-enterprise:

> "When she comes in sometimes and she says 'you look tired', you know she does notice and I say 'oh no, I'm fine', and she does realise, the support is there for us really." (Carer 222, Micro day service)

These examples relate to the support given by micro-enterprises. In day centre services, some carers also reported feeling more supported by the larger settings. In the next example, where support comes from a large day centre, the carer again talked about benefits both for the person receiving the support and for herself.

> "I know it's benefitted her because when I come to collect her it's my most favourite time of the week because for a brief time I've got my mum back. When I come to pick her up she's bright, alert, bubbly, she'll be chatting all the way home in the car, you know, 'what we having for tea, I'm hungry', which shows me as well she's been using her brain during the day, you know, cos she's hungry, it's the mental – she's been using, burning that energy up, using her brain. Goes away after about an hour, you know, after you've got her home. Yeah, she gets back into her habits, but for that hour it's lovely." (Carer 327, Large day service)

The same theme, of a relationship being restored, is also evident in this example, drawn from the sister of someone who had recently started receiving support from a medium-sized accommodation day service:

> "[W]e do leisurely things like sisters can do instead of doing all the cooking and her washing and bathing her and things like that. The support people help her with that, so we have a more leisurely connection now, you know." (Carer 233, Medium day service)

In all of these examples the well-being of the family carer is enhanced both through the practical help that the care agency or day centre provides, which frees up their time to do other things, and also through the trust that they have in the provider, which enables them to relax and enjoy that time. For home care this level of trust was strongest when care was provided by the micro-enterprises; for day centres, the experience did not follow a pattern of size of provider, and some carers reported positive outcomes for themselves when the person they cared for was in a large day centre setting.

Positive experiences of large day centres are somewhat counter-cultural in an era in which building-based services have often been seeing as lying outside the personalisation narrative (for a discussion see Needham, 2014). Large day centres have been subject to critique from a range of advocates of personalised approaches for taking a 'warehousing' approach to support for older people and people with disabilities (Leadbeater, 2004; Cottam, 2009; Duffy, 2010). The more positive experiences of the family carers reported here run counter to that. In the next chapter, we discuss some positive aspects of large day centres in relation to personalisation. It is apposite here to note, though, that outcomes for family carers and the person being cared for need not always be aligned (Needham, 2011). Following a history of invisibility, family carers have gained increased attention in recent social care reforms, gaining equal legal recognition with the person being cared for, following the passage of the Care Act 2014. Carers are entitled to an assessment and to 'maintain a balance between their caring responsibilities and a life outside caring' (HM Government, 2008, p 9). They may themselves be eligible for a personal budget. However, it is not necessarily the case that the models of service provision that carers prefer will be those preferred by the person receiving support. A potential weakness of our study is that some family carers were interviewed along with the person they were supporting, which inhibited the potential for different perspectives on the service to emerge.

Value for money

Having considered, in the first half of the chapter, the extent to which micro-enterprises and larger care organisations are able to achieve valued outcomes for the people that they support, the chapter now goes on to discuss the extent to which the case study organisations offer good value for money. Price data from the 27 organisations in the research study was used to assess how the hourly unit prices in micro-enterprises differ from those of larger providers. It is important to note that the study includes only organisations that have a trading income, that is, they charge for their services. Many statutory services, charities and social enterprises work on a voluntary basis and are free for disabled and older people using them, but they are not included in this research. The discussion below considers pricing data, but also highlights the need to interpret this data by considering how care is paid for and what relevant differences are collapsed by discussing care as a unit of one hour of support.

We opted to use pricing data as the basis of comparison rather than cost data. It is common in social policy to use expenditure measures based on unit costs for comparative research (PSSRU, 2010). However, the move to personalisation within social care has been accompanied by a call to providers to restructure their business models to utilise prices for personal budget holders rather than costs for local authority block purchasers (ACEVO, 2010). By using pricing here, it is not possible to assess whether smaller organisations use inputs more efficiently than larger ones. A focus on pricing does, however, have compelling advantages.

- Relevance: price is the financial variable that service users, carers and public bodies use to compare services.
- Transparency: price is a publicly available measure, whereas organisations may not release costing information where it is considered to be covered by commercial confidentiality.
- Simplicity: price facilitates comparison between organisations with different legal forms and staffing models.

During the staff interviews we gathered price data from all of the 27 organisations included in the research (17 micros, 4 small, 4 medium and 2 large organisations). Using the hourly charge – rather than the daily rate or charge per home visit – enhanced the comparability of the findings across different types of care provider. Hourly rate was the price unit that providers most frequently gave us when we asked about their charges. Analysis of the hourly pricing data from the case study organisations indicated that micro–enterprises were slightly cheaper in their hourly rate than small, medium and large care providers (Figure 6.1).

Figure: 6.1: Hourly prices for care providers, by size

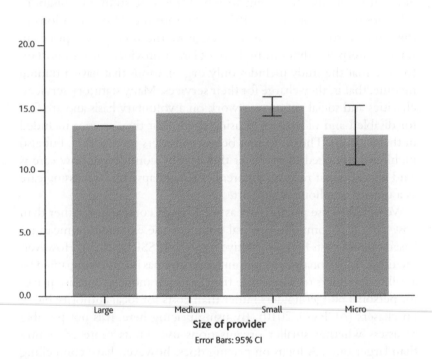

Size of provider

Error Bars: 95% CI

When compared to the average price of home care in England (by councils and external providers), micro–enterprises remained cheaper at £12.80 per hour, as compared to £14 by external providers and £29 for council-run services (Table 6.2).

The relatively small sample size (particularly for the small, medium and large providers) means that we cannot generalise from this to say that micro-enterprises are always cheaper. However, it does indicate that economies-of-scale arguments do not necessarily hold in a linear way within the care sector, at least not in terms of hourly prices: the larger organisations in our study were rarely able to offer a service at a lower hourly rate than a comparable micro-enterprise, although the largest organisations were cheaper than the small and medium organisations. Again, it is difficult to generalise from such a small sample, but from

Table 6.2: Comparing average hourly prices of care

	Average hourly cost of care
National (council-provided care)	£29
National (non-council provider)	£14
Micro	£12.80
Small	£15.10
Medium	£14.50
Large	£13.60

Note: National data is based on average cost to purchase one hour of home-based care in England (data from HSCIC, 2015).

what we observed through interviews with these organisations it appeared that small and medium providers face a particularly difficult financial context. They don't have the economies of scale of the large organisations, and they also don't have the low overheads of the micro-enterprises, most of which worked out of their homes or very small office spaces and employed few if any staff. This supports findings from the CQC *State of Care Report 2015*, which reported that, in a highly challenging financial context, medium-sized providers were closing and growth was coming from new, large providers (CQC, 2015, p 17).

We also examined the relationship between hourly price and valued outcomes (as derived from ASCOT) for micro-enterprises and larger organisations. Our findings indicated that micro-enterprises delivered better outcomes (as discussed in the previous section) for a lower average hourly price than large providers. Therefore, those using cheaper services had more control and did more things they valued and enjoyed, as compared with those using more expensive care services (Figures 6.2 and 6.3). Furthermore, comparing the costs of the individual organisations showed that for the micro-enterprises there was an inverse relationship between outcomes and price (so outcomes were better when services were cheaper), while for larger services outcomes remained fairly consistent, regardless of price. While this may mean that a higher price tag does not lead to better outcomes, these findings do need to be interpreted with caution, as people using micro-enterprises may have lower levels of need in the first place. The small sample size also needs restating as a limitation.

The headline findings about the relatively low prices charged by micro-enterprises do also need to be contextualised so as to be sensitive to the different types of service offered, and the different ways in

Figure 6.2: 'Doing things I value and enjoy', by price and organisational size

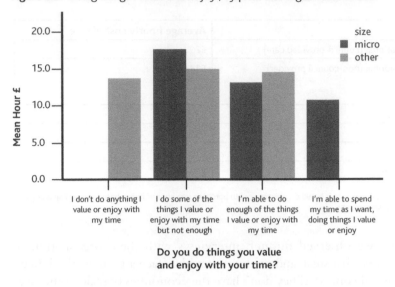

Do you do things you value
and enjoy with your time?

Figure 6.3: 'Having choice and control', by price and organisational size

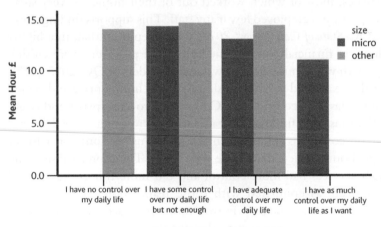

Do you feel you have control
over your daily life?

which care is paid for. These contextual factors are discussed below. In Chapter Ten we discuss the relationship between care providers and the local authority and the extent to which this impacts on how much they can charge and how financially sustainable they are likely to be.

What happens in an hour?

In contextualising this hourly pricing data, it is important to note that many of the providers we spoke to did not actually work in hour chunks. Day services were usually available for longer periods. Domiciliary care was often divided into smaller time periods. The largest domiciliary organisation in the sample offered 15-minute visits, and it was through these short visits that they were able to offer the local authority a lower rate than the micro-enterprises would charge. When providing domiciliary care, the micro-enterprises (and indeed some of the small providers) would only undertake calls of 30 minutes or longer, making them more expensive to commission per visit than a company operating on a 15-minutes-per-call basis. One of the micro-enterprises we interviewed felt that his organisation was struggling to compete on price with the larger providers.

> "We could only drop our prices if we multiplied our business by a factor of five or six. And put, you know, volume into it. Then there's economies of scale. But at the levels we're running at, we can't." (Staff 103, Micro domiciliary care)

The longer calls offered by micro-providers were in part driven by practicality, given the small staff base and the difficulties of moving staff to a different location after 15 minutes. For some of the smaller organisations it was also a matter of ethos.

> "They're given 15-minute calls or, you know, a very short amount of time where you can't value somebody and respect them. So I decided that I wouldn't do anything less than 30 minutes. If it's personal care I won't do anything less than an hour. I'd rather not have a business than do something that isn't right." (Staff 310, Small domiciliary care)

The large domiciliary care company in our sample was required to offer 15-minute visits as part of its framework agreement with the local authority. It is important to note that this company also recognised the problems of the 15-minute model, particularly from a staff perspective: "[the local authority] do the 15-minute visits which staff don't want to do" (Staff 113, Large domiciliary care). Working across two local authorities, one of which required 15 minutes, whereas the other commissioned a minimum of 30-minute visits, the large company was clear that it preferred to work with the longer approach.

This point affirms what is known from the secondary literature: that 15-minute visits are not popular with staff or with the people using services. Research indicates that 15 minutes is not long enough to provide good-quality care and such narrow time constraints deprive people of their dignity and act as a barrier to the development of good relations between people who use the service and the care worker (Leonard Cheshire, 2013; Walsh and Shutes, 2013; NICE, 2015). The organisation Locality has argued that 'bulk buying support, at scale and at rock bottom prices' (Locality, 2014, p 8) leads to diseconomies of scale, as failure demand must be managed: 'Counterintuitively, mass-produced poor service is more costly than personalised service that meets individual need' (Locality, 2014, p 39). Although it is beyond the scope of our study, this does link to broader concerns that pressures on acute hospital services and on family carers are intensified by the time-and-task approach to mass-produced care (Leonard Cheshire, 2013). There has been a national emphasis on eradicating 15-minute care visits, which are offered by around three-quarters of local authorities, although in fact they may be becoming more prevalent again as a response to cuts in care funding (UNISON, 2014; NICE, 2015). The commitment that micro-enterprises and some small providers in our sample made to rejecting the 15-minute model therefore can be seen as in line with national understandings of what constitutes good care.

Who pays for the care and support?

The ways in which people can pay for their care funding are also a relevant factor in exploring pricing data. Care services are means tested, as well as needs tested, so people cannot receive state-funded services unless their assets fall below a nationally established threshold. People near the threshold may find that they have to make some contribution to their care costs, in addition to partial state funding. For people whose care is all or partly state funded, there are three main options: they can have that service commissioned by the local authority, they can have a personal budget managed for them by the local authority or third party, or the money can come to them (or their family) as a direct payment. People who pay most or all of their care costs themselves are usually referred to as self-funders. Exact numbers of self-funders are unknown because not all of them make contact with local authorities and some home care operates as informal private domestic help (Henwood, 2014, p 76). Estimates of self-funding levels are around 45% in residential care and around 20% in home care (IPC, 2011). Better support for and tracking of self-funders is one of the themes of the Care Act 2014.

Micro-enterprises generally cannot be paid for through traditional forms of commissioning or managed personal budgets because local authority procurement processes are ill-adapted to contracting with very small firms. The people in our study who used micro-enterprises were predominantly paying for them through direct payments or as self-funders. This is an important factor to bear in mind when comparing them with larger providers, who were more likely to be delivering services commissioned by the local authority. This potentially distorts the comparison between micro- and larger providers in two ways. The first is that people on direct payments – still a minority of eligible people and predominantly concentrated in younger people with disabilities rather than older people – may be those with better networks and more personal efficacy than those who are not (Slasberg et al, 2012a, 2012b). These factors are likely to be linked to a greater propensity to deviate from local authority-recommended provider lists and find their own support services that are better tailored to their individual needs. Certainly in our interviews, direct payments were almost entirely used by people with learning disabilities: most older people had a managed personal budget or were self-funders, with only one direct payment holder.

In all three localities the costs of care were shaped by the hourly rate that the local authority was willing to pay for the care services that it funded. Most of the larger providers situated themselves exactly at this rate, since the majority of their care work was generated by local authority referrals – although they charged a higher rate to self-funders. Many of the micro-providers offered a slightly lower rate than the local authority rate, partly reflecting their low overheads. However, it also came from an effort to be competitive in an environment in which they sought to get more referrals from the local authority. Some found that this competitiveness was still not enough, because the local authority expected them to compete with the personal assistant rate rather than the standard care provider rate, and this was generally a few pounds less per hour.

> "I charge £11.50 an hour for specialist work. But the council don't want to pay [personal assistants] any more than £10 an hour and then they top-slice money off that to pay for brokerage even if brokerage isn't needed. So I don't always get £11.50 an hour ... So sometimes I will settle for £10 or £8 an hour because there's two rates

... And nobody can tell me why and nobody can tell me how the pricing works ... And then of course I'm not – I don't have the same job security in a big company now. If I put my head above the parapet that's me gone." (Staff 206, Micro day service)

The small and medium providers often priced themselves slightly above the local authority rate, reflecting their higher overheads and lack of economics of scale. They tended to have a higher proportion of self-funders, in comparison to the large providers. One of the most expensive organisations in the study, a small provider whose higher prices meant that it too was excluded from the local authority's preferred provider framework, had found a distinctive space in the market as a high-price, high-quality offer for self-funders.

This point affirms the complex relationship between price and quality for different categories of people. Economic theory, and the example above, might suggest that self-funders can find a price point where they get the quality that they want. However, price and quality in the care market do not operate in this way. Self-funders (that is, the more affluent people in an area) generally pay more for care than the local authority pays for the people it funds, even when receiving exactly the same service. This cross-subsidisation is well known in the residential care sector (IPC, 2011). Self-funders have been found to struggle to use their purported market power to secure a good-quality service (Henwood, 2010). A report on self-funders by Henwood noted that 'For some people there was a profound sense of "powerlessness" and lack of control over their own financial resources, coupled with some real fear over what would become of them if their savings ran dry ... It is clear that having sufficient resources to be a self-funder does not automatically give people greater control over their situation, and meaningful choices are often lacking' (Henwood, 2010, pp 48, 50).

In the context of micro-enterprises, what being a self-funder offered the people that we interviewed seemed to be two-fold: firstly, the scope to access services at a lower level of need (for example, getting someone in to provide help around the home and in getting out and about in the community); secondly, the potential to use the time more flexibly, adding on extra bits of support on a more ad hoc basis (for example, to go to an evening social event, or get help with some DIY). Direct payment holders similarly also have some flexibility to use the service in a way that meets fluctuating need and to make decisions about how much to pay for a particular service, although this may be limited in practice by what overall financial allocation they have been given.

For people whose care is purchased for them by the local authority, the cost/quality trade-offs are hidden from them but are much more intense, since they can access only those services that can be delivered at the local authority rate. Local authorities have been required to cut social care by 25% percent in since 2014, with more cuts likely in the future. With a rising population of older people who need care, they are likely to feel that they have little choice but to continue to place downward pressure on prices and to chunk care up into brief visits (LGA, 2015).

Attempts to find a more satisfactory model of funding care so as to bring sufficient money into the sector have so far failed to address the cost/quality trade-offs for people funded by the local authority and the patchy experience of self-funders (Commission on Funding of Care and Support, 2011). The cap on care costs contained in the Care Act 2014 could potentially help self-funders (although only a small minority, because of the high level of the cap). However, it is likely to intensify rather than reduce spending pressures on local authorities, and, after campaigning by the Local Government Association (LGA), implementation has been delayed until 2020. The absence of public and political will to fund care services on a level equivalent to health places a major strain on all care providers, including micro-enterprises. The LGA has estimated that the large-scale cuts to care services, triggered by the broader public sector austerity, have led to a £700 million annual shortfall between the money available and what is needed (LGA, 2015).

Conclusion

This chapter has presented research findings in relation to two of the hypotheses underpinning the research: that micro-enterprises achieve more valued outcomes and better value for money than larger care providers. The chapter began with a discussion of care outcomes, arguably the 'fool's gold' of contemporary public policy. The ASCOT tool was used to gather outcomes data during the project, which has the advantage of being a validated and widely used tool within social care. Findings from ASCOT highlighted the strong performance of micro-enterprises on the two domains that were measured (doing things I value with my time; having choice and control). Comparing the findings to the national ASCOT data also showed a strong relative scoring for micro-enterprises, although only the 'doing things I value with my time' was statistically significant. The second part of the chapter considered the extent to which such organisations offer value for money. It focused on the hourly rate in relation to the outcomes data outlined earlier in the chapter, and concluded that, when set alongside the outcomes data, micro-enterprises do offer value for money.

It is important also to discuss the contextual factors that need to be taken into account when interpreting this headline finding. Who buys care and how is one key factor, with the local authority playing a significant role in shaping the care market. The type of care being provided is also a relevant factor, with the standardised measure of an hour not necessarily capturing effectively the differences in provision between short chunks of domiciliary care and much longer stints at a day service. The financial context within which micro-enterprises operate, and the extent to which the broader policy, market and regulatory contexts enable micro-enterprises to be financially viable, is another factor to consider. We discuss this issue more in Chapter Ten in relation to the sustainability of micro care providers.

SEVEN

Enacting personalisation on a micro scale

This chapter and the next seek to examine what is in the 'black box' of the outcome data – focusing on the process of care as a key element in explaining how good care outcomes are attained. Here research findings are presented about how far the micro-enterprises are more person-centred than larger providers. The main data source for the discussion of personalisation is interviews with the people who use services, family carers and staff.

Interest in the process of public service delivery is coming back into fashion within public management, as the journey from outputs to outcomes has been felt to neglect a focus on the interpersonal aspects of the care process in social and medical settings. The avoidable deaths of hundreds of patients at Mid-Staffordshire NHS Foundation Trust were found to have been in part due to failings at the interpersonal level, with a focus on meeting financial and performance targets eclipsing compassionate care to patients (Francis, 2012). Interpersonal relationships are particularly important in the close and sometimes private settings in which care and support are provided.

Literature that explores care services in the context of an ethic of care is proliferating (for example Barnes, 2012; Lewis and West, 2014; Barnes et al, 2015). In some ways, argue Lewis and West (2014, p 3) this marks a revival of the 1980s feminist literature that:

> questioned the idea that care work could ever be 'reduced' to tending, or, later, to 'tasks' such as bathing, feeding and toileting, that could be commodified (Ungerson, 1983, 1987; Lewis and Meredith, 1989). 'Caring about' the person-cared-for was conceptualised as an integral part of carework, involving compassion and kindness, which cannot be legislated for or commodified. Most importantly, these authors emphasised that 'the care relationship' was crucial to the experience of care.

To better understand the process of care, the relationships that underpinned it and the relevance of organisational size within that, we used the qualitative interview data to analyse the interactions between people who use services and the paid workers who provide their care and support.

Defining personalised support

As discussed in Chapter Two, the term personalisation came to prominence in English social care services around 2007, and has been interpreted in various different ways (Needham, 2011; Needham and Glasby, 2014). It usually refers to a sense that services are tailored to the individual: as Carr puts it, personalisation requires 'thinking about public services ... in an entirely different way – starting with the person rather than the service' (Carr, 2010, p 67). However, beyond this broad insight, its implementation across different local authorities has proceeded very differently (Ellis, 2015).

Despite being an extensively analysed and debated policy, personalisation itself has been under-theorised. What it means to be personalised is usually presented in tautologous terms as centred on the person, or else illustrated through individual vignettes of transformative change. We used the interview data to get a sense of what it means for personalisation to be enacted: what are the types of behaviour or relationships that embody person–centredness. Enactment is used in the sense that Weick (1988, p 306) defined: 'when people act, they bring events and structures into existence and set them in motion'. Here we focus then on personalisation being brought into existence.

We asked the people being interviewed about how they had come to be using the particular support service that they were, what support was provided, how much choice there was about the service and who provided it, and what kind of relationship they had with the people providing it. The examples that people gave in response to these interview questions were of course all very place- and person-specific. In the first phase of coding, we categorised together everything that seemed to exemplify person–centred care. In the second, inductive phase of coding, we identified four different themes in the data on what it meant for services to be personalised.

a) Care providers are willing to be flexible and spontaneous about the sort of support that is offered at a particular encounter.
b) Care providers anticipate the needs of individuals.
c) Care providers act in a way more akin to being a family member or a friend.

d) Care providers allow individuals to have choice and control in relation to their activities or support.

Personalisation as types (a)–(c) seemed to be particularly important to the activities that went on in people's homes (that is, domiciliary care and the more generic one-to-one support). In group day activities, personalisation as type (d) was the most often invoked. This fits with the notion of the home as a distinctive private space in which intimate 'body work' is undertaken and different sorts of interpersonal engagement are appropriate (Twigg, 2000). This sense that the home is somehow different was exemplified by this quote from a family carer:

> "You just got the feeling that it was a very personalised service and that was really nice because at the end of the day, they're in my mum's home and they're her primary carers so you have to kind of feel that they are interested." (Carer 331, Small domiciliary care)

From the data, we concluded that there were aspects of micro-enterprises' provision that did allow them to offer a more personalised service than larger providers, particularly for care and support that is delivered within the home. Small organisations also performed well on this measure, whereas medium and large organisations did less well. For day activities, the difference between organisations of different sizes was less clear: there were several examples of micro-enterprises offering highly personalised day activities, but we also found examples of larger providers offering greater choice. Below we look at examples of personalisation as types (a)–(d) in more detail to draw out these points.

Flexibility and spontaneity

A criticism of care services has been the tendency to take a time and task approach, in which care-related activities are highly specified and narrow in scope, in ways that limit the potential to be flexible to the needs and preferences of the person needing support (Lewis and West, 2014).

A staff member from a micro-enterprise explained her willingness to deviate from the set task:

> "All I do, supposed to do is supposed to cook. When I'm there if she wants her nails doing I'll paint her nails or wash

her hair and set it, whatever they want to do really." (Staff 109, Micro one-to-one support)

One of the people receiving services from a micro-enterprise explained the flexibility of what was provided:

> "She's having a go at painting this [wall], she hasn't finished it yet … I call her 'Odd Job' I do because there ain't much she can't do, she's a smasher of a girl, really is." (Older person 120, Micro one-to-one support)

An interviewee running a small day service highlighted the desire to be as spontaneous as possible:

> "I'm really very anxious that we … don't even think it's like the old statutory services where Monday it was craft, Tuesday it was IT, Wednesday it was this, Thursday it was this and then people sat around almost like an old folk's home. So I think because we're small and flexible, you know, if people say 'well actually I don't want to do that, let's go and do such and such', and we can say 'well what about going outside' and 'what about going to the park today' so I think we can have that flexibility because numbers are smaller." (Staff 205, Micro day service)

Most of these examples were from micro-enterprises, although one of the small providers also drew praise for its flexible approach to care tasks:

> *Older person:* "I was expecting them to just come in and do the necessary, but the first thing they did was to smarten my hair up.
> *Family carer:* "And it brightened you up no end." (Older person and carer 130, Small domiciliary care)

This point about flexible use of time maps most closely onto the ASCOT domain, which showed that micro-enterprises were more likely than larger care providers to score well in terms of people being able to do what they valued and enjoyed with their time. While our analysis did not find many examples of people complaining about the narrowness of tasks done by the larger providers, there was a relative absence of positive examples of flexible and responsive services similar to those given above.

Anticipating needs

A second theme of person-centredness related to the ability of the care worker to anticipate the needs of the person being cared for. One interviewee contrasted the support that she used to get from two of her previous providers – one a small provider and the second a large provider – which affirms the importance of staff continuity and personal relationships:

> "When I used to have [a previous Small care provider] she knew where to get my cream out and get this and that, put it away and get a clean towel if there wasn't one out, you know. She used to do all that, no problems at all. That lot [from a large care agency] they just look at you." (Older person 319, Small one-to-one support)

The following extracts from interviews with people using micro and small services articulate an appreciation of having someone who anticipates their needs.

> "Well that day I was watching the Armistice and all that sort of thing. And she knows me inside out. She said you've been crying. And she come switched the telly off." (Older person 317, Small domiciliary care)

> "I give her my shopping list and she goes down and she'll say 'Do you want so and so? Do you want butter? Salt?' or whatever, but she'll go down it and certain things I don't need to mention because she knows I want them. I don't put them down she'll say 'You haven't got so and so down' because she's used to doing it." (Older person 319, Small one-to-one support)

> "She put [mum] a note on the calendar to say, you know, when Deal or No Deal's on." (Carer 103, Micro one-to-one support)

These examples seemed to us to be enactments of person-centredness, illustrations of the sorts of relationships that people wanted from their carers. Not all of these came from micro-enterprises: some were small care providers. We did not get any comparable examples from the medium and large providers.

Akin to family member or friend

A third enactment of personalised care provided by the smaller organisations in the study was the sense of an almost familial bond with the person being supported. One person running a small domiciliary care agency put it in the following terms:

> "They just resemble your Nan. You just do things for them as you would for your own parents, family." (Staff 112, Small domiciliary care)

Talking about friendship, a family carer said:

> "And, yeah, they didn't wear uniforms either, that was the other thing we quite liked about it, they came in their own clothes and very much blended into the home environment, you know, and they became friends and that was very obvious, that was the huge difference I think, that they were very, very good friends with my mum and they even want to go and see her now [she is in a residential care home], you see, which I don't think you would get in a lot of organisations and that's what I liked." (Carer 129, Small domiciliary care)

Within day services, this sense of familiarity was invoked in relation to the environment being more like a home than an institution. This person running a micro day service describes her efforts to create a home-like environment:

> "I went to a social service [day service] and it was enormous and I felt that the people were lost within the building ... I just felt that it was not personal ... all the chairs were in lines around the edge of the room ... All a bit clinical, I didn't like it, it didn't seem like homely and friendly, so that to me was not good. Whereas here it's like somebody's front room because it's bigger than that but it's not too big, so it's quite personal and we can really get to know people properly." (Staff 105, Micro day service)

In this next example, an older person looked to the micro provider rather than her family as the first point of contact in an emergency:

> "I wasn't very well because I had a nose bleed a couple of nights ago and I don't usually get that, but it lasted and lasted. And [the care provider] was having an evening off which she never does very often and so [I phoned her] and said oh I don't know what to do. So she got straight in touch with my son and his wife and they came round and they stayed with me. So it was alright." (Older person 101, Micro one-to-one support)

Contacting the care provider rather than the family first, despite the worker's having an 'evening off' highlights some of the potential tensions in this more familial type of relationship. There is scope for a blurring of boundaries between formal support and friendship that can create problems of over-attachment or unprofessionalism. One family carer reflected on his uncertainty about whether or not the people providing care for his spouse were allowed to talk about personal issues:

> "[The micro provider] talks about her family and sometimes when the grandchildren are here [the provider] might be here and they chat. So they, they do get involved with the families ... I don't know whether people in the training stress objectivity and say you should remove yourself a little bit, but I find that getting involved helps a lot more." (Carer 124, Micro one-to-one support)

The boundary between objectivity and 'getting involved' was one that seemed particularly porous in relation to micro-enterprises. We did not come across any cases where relationships had crossed boundaries to such an extent that we felt there were safeguarding concerns. However, some people we interviewed had encountered problems around informal types of relationship. One person using services explained that a one-to-one support worker employed by the local authority had got into trouble for being perceived to transgress boundaries:

> "Yeah because with [the staff member] we went out and stuff and then he stopped working, like his work hours had finished and we went out for a drink and he got in trouble for that, they said it's a conflict of interest. He said 'yeah, but I'm his friend as well', because he is." (Person with learning disability 223, Micro day service)

We had assumed that people using the services and family carers would want the service to be as personalised as possible – whereas staff or managers would be the ones putting the brakes on the development of close relationships (as in the example above). However, some family carers were also concerned that over-attachment could occur. As one interviewee put it, talking about her daughter,

> "[S]he doesn't like one person coming all the time cos obviously they can get an attachment, can't they? Then, if for whatever reason they're not able to come then, you know, you've got a fresh face, whereas if there's a few people bobbing in and out they get to know that person, aren't they, over the time and know their ways and what they've got to do and where things are." (Carer 328, Small one-to-one support)

Another person receiving services also talked of the benefits of having more than one person providing support to a family member, having been supported by a PA in the past:

> "[I]f you just had a PA you just see that person and it gets very, you can get very sort of attached, it's like a marriage really, if somebody is coming in in the morning and at night … Whereas if you've got three people coming in or four people, whatever, at least you've got a selective amount of people and you can have a chat with them." (Carer 107, Micro domiciliary care)

This point, although coming from only one interviewee, reinforces much of the literature on PAs, in which boundaries were found to be hard to maintain (Spandler, 2004; Yeandle and Stiell, 2007; Leece 2010; Leece and Peace, 2010). Micro-enterprises, supporting a number of people rather than just one, may be able to offer person-centredness without the emotional intensity of the PA relationship. However, there is scope for over-attachment and uncertain boundaries in the sole-trader model, which some people felt uncomfortable about.

Choice and control

The fourth enactment of personalised care was that people felt that they had choice and control over the support provided. The ASCOT data highlighted that more people using micro-enterprises felt that they had choice and control than those using larger providers, although the differences were not statistically significant. Using the interview data to interrogate the dimensions of choice and control further showed that these two concepts – so often run together in the personalisation policy literature and in the ASCOT domain itself – need disaggregating. Although both of these terms are vague enough to be defined in ways that are synonymous, this seems to lose the relevant difference between them. In relation to home care services, what people seemed to crave was some control and predictability, rather than anything that could accurately be called choice. It was clear that some of the larger home care services performed poorly on this measure, as the following quotes indicate, in which both interviewees talk about previous experiences with a large domiciliary care service:

> "You see when you've got carers coming like they did latterly at four times a day, you've no control at all. You've just got to work with them, you know, when they come you've got to, you know you're going to be there. You've not gone anywhere. And they don't come for any length of time to let you go out." (Older person 314, Small domiciliary care service)

> "I've never been given a time. They can come anytime in the morning, they can come and bang on the bedroom window at quarter to seven to half past eleven. They come for a bath, you know when they come for my bath, it will always be half past eleven when they come. And you're sat here with dressing gown on and nightie. And then one of them said 'don't know why you don't have a key safe'. Well I said I would do but I don't want people walking in my house at that time of the morning, it would frighten me." (Older person 319, Small one-to-one support)

In relation to day services, it was the quite different concept of choice of activities that was most commonly brought up by interviewees. Here, larger day services seemed as likely as smaller ones to be able to have a positive impact. When it came to activities outside the home, some interviewees argued that a larger scale enabled more diversity of provision and therefore potentially a better responsiveness to individualised need.

Larger day centres were usually able to provide a greater range of activities each day, including, for example baking, mood rooms, computer rooms, music activities, drama groups, arts and crafts. One provider, which runs a large day service, suggested that the bustle of a large, busy day centre was what people came for. When the numbers of people using the service had dropped at weekends, "gradually [people] started to transfer into the week because it was boring because there wasn't enough people about. They couldn't, you know there was one activity basically because there was one room" (Staff 307, Large day service).

A family carer also preferred the larger-scale day provision, because of the broader range of choice on offer:

> "I think because it is bigger there's lots of different activities, so there's more there to interest the people that come here. Whereas if you're in a smaller place they could probably only do a handful of activities at any time, so some people might not be want to go and do the cooking or go and do the flower arranging or whatever it is that they're doing." (Carer 327, Large day service)

The large day services in our sample showed examples where they were able to offer more choice of activities, while micro-enterprises offering day activities were more targeted in their approach, matching activities to the interests and needs of the people in the centre each day on a more ad hoc basis. Box 7.1 shows the different kinds of offer provided by very small and much larger day services.

Box 7.1: Comparing micro and large day activities

Micro-enterprise day support

Small Steps day service is a micro-enterprise employing two members of staff and providing a community-based day service for older people. The service supports approximately 10 people a day and runs a range of activities tailored to whoever is in the centre that day. The owner explains its approach:

> "I think we offer a more personable service for people, especially for the carers ... they talk to us and you know they see us hopefully as, I wouldn't say friends but you know, somebody that they can trust ... one lady came with her husband for the first time cos he'd got Alzheimer's and he wasn't sort of settling in places. And she was helping wash the pots and that and she just broke down in tears. She said 'I'm so glad I've found somewhere that, somebody that I can talk to'." (Staff 302, Micro day service)

Large day support

Sunnyville Day Centre is a large local authority day service and supports over 100 people a day. People who attend include older people, people with learning disabilities and people with physical disabilities. It offers a range of activities every day, enabling people to tailor their activities according to their needs and interests.

> "We offer a choice of things to do on each day ... the coffee bar ...we have a hair salon and our therapy room we'll do foot massages, nails, beauty sort of stuff, so there's that side ... we need to be offering lots of different styles of things to motivate people or make people feel nice about their selves and feel cared for. So we do lots of beauty therapies, lots of foot massage. We've got a Reiki Master and she does Reiki with some people, hair, make-up. Then we have art and craft sessions, card making sessions, cookery, basic cookery ... We have sports, we have chair keep fit and stuff like that and you know, karaoke, sing-alongs, bingo." (Staff 307, Large day service)

Overall, then, micro–enterprises performed well on the personalisation dimension, offering person-centred support in a number of different ways. The data allowed us to draw out four enactments of personalisation and to highlight the ways in which different sizes of organisation supported these enactments. Micro and small organisations were best able to contribute to most of these types of personalisation, although large organisations performed well in terms of choice of activities.

Why are micro-enterprises more personalised?

Having identified four enactments of personalisation, it is important to explain why most of these appear to be found more in micro–enterprises than in larger providers. While larger providers of day services sometimes provided more choice of services, which some people liked, on the whole the micro and small providers performed better on the other aspects of being personalised, relating to being more flexible, anticipating need and being more like a friend of family. These were particularly important to people in the services they received in their homes.

In the second phase of coding of the data, we looked for attributes of the micro-enterprises that might explain their tendency to behave in more personalised ways. We found that the more personalised care provided by the smaller-scale providers in the home was attributed by interviewees to three aspects of their approach:

- autonomy of front-line staff to vary the service being offered
- continuity of front-line staff, as compared to large care providers
- accessibility of managers to front-line staff and people using the service.

Autonomy

The first of these – the *autonomy* of front-line staff – was demonstrated in interviews with people running micro-enterprises and people using the services, where care and support was defined in very flexible terms. The 'time and task' model is well known (and much criticised) as the dominant approach to domiciliary care delivery, denoting very short care visits to undertake highly specified tasks (Equality and Human Rights Commission, 2011). This model was one that the staff in the micro-enterprises and the small organisations define themselves in opposition to:

> "Being a small company … you don't have to be so task driven. This is the list of things that we're supposed to do on the care plan for whoever, but when you go in if you can see that they're down and they need you to sit and have a cup of tea with them. You know, that's absolutely fine. 'Cause you wouldn't go and visit your mother and your mother's looking like, you know devastated about something, and just start hoovering or ironing, would you? You wouldn't do it would you?" (Staff 310, Small domiciliary care)

One micro-provider providing a one-to-one support service as a sole trader explained how she had gone into someone's home to provide a meals service, and then went further than that because of the perceived need:

> "Took this new man on. Dementia. It was a, like, holiday cover. His sister's gone away. [She] says, 'Will just go and, you know, do his dinner for me? Just put the vac round?' He's got a dog. 'Cause he's got dementia, every time the dog barks, he feeds him. So he's just barking all the while, so he's just giving the dog food. And [his sister] says, 'Just do his dinner and go.' So now, what I do, put his dinner in

when I get there, wash up, wipe the sides down, put it on the plate, put the vac round, and when that's cooled down, give him his dinner and take the dog a walk. Stops the dog barking and he can eat his dinner in peace. And he's ate at least three-quarters of his dinner every day." (Staff 101, Micro one-to-one support)

In each of these cases staff had the autonomy to make an adjustment during the care encounter rather than being limited to a prior specification.

Staff in both the micro and small organisations framed their distinctive offer in terms of their more personal connection with people using the service, and also with staff:

"I've not come across anything yet that I've asked [service provider] and she's said, 'No, we can't do that.' Do you know what I mean? So they'll stand and do a bit of my mum's ironing and chat to her and just engage in conversation with her really. Which is what I want, I want them to talk to her and be in the house and be company as well as doing care. I think that's the more important thing so I'm happy if I go in and they're sat on the settee and they're chatting to my mum, that's fine." (Carer 331, Small domiciliary care)

One person remembered the inflexibility of a large provider (whom she no longer uses) immediately after the death of her husband. She called the agency to ask if for one week following her husband's death they could call earlier than her normal 10:30am slot. She describes the phone call:

"And I heard [the manager] saying, she said you can tell [the service user] her time's half past ten and not a minute before. And do you know for two days after that it was half past eleven when they came." (Older person 319, Small one-to-one support)

Box 7.2 gives an example of a micro-enterprise offering personalised care and support. John's approach and the satisfaction reported by the people using the service highlight the potential for micro-enterprises to perform well on the personalisation measure. However, we return to this example in Chapter Nine, because by the time the research project was nearing completion John informed us that he would no longer continue trading because he couldn't make the organisation financially sustainable, underscoring the fragility of the micro-enterprise sector.

Box 7.2: Personalised care and support on a micro scale

John set up his micro-enterprise My Support four years ago. He had worked in the IT departments of large care agencies and has over 20 years of experience as a family carer. As he puts it, "as a parent [of a child with autism] as a purchaser of services and also purchasing services for two elderly relatives ... I thought, I can do better than this. I can certainly do it different and more person-centred." His agency grew through local advertising and word-of-mouth recommendations until it was supporting 12 people. His stated aim was to be able to offer everyone a service that he would want for his mum and his son. This included breakfast at a reasonable hour, and care that was consistent and high quality. Visits are for a minimum of 30 minutes, as John didn't believe that good-quality support could be offered in a shorter time. The people whom we interviewed who used John's company rate the service very highly. As one put it:

"I think because they're a smaller organisation they've got control on their staff and I have rotas sent through to me by e-mail regularly and then or they get in touch with me by text and say 'oh it won't be so and so tonight because they've had to juggle it round and it's such and such'. They've got more control on the staff and what they're doing ... they haven't got too many clients ... they're very selective in who they provide the care for." (Carer 107, Micro domiciliary care).

Continuity

The second aspect of the personalised offer from micro-enterprises was that they offered *continuity* of staffing. For people using micro-enterprises, this was the key aspect that they drew out:

"I think it's quite nice. It's small cos you're not gonna get loads of different people coming, are you? (Older person 328, Micro domiciliary care)

The number of different staff coming in from large agencies was reported by interviewees as being higher than for the micro-enterprises. In one case, a family carer whose spouse was supported by a large care provider felt the numbers to be extremely high:

> *Interviewer:* When [the carers] come, is it normally – how many different people would you get? Is it normally the same one or two, or could it be a lot?
> *Respondent:* Oh it could be dozens, because there's that many. (Carer 132, Large domiciliary care)

Another family carer set the number lower but still felt troubled by the lack of continuity presented by the staff team at the large agency:

> *Interviewer:* How many different people do you have coming in?
> *Respondent:* Six ... And it's getting me down. (Carer 133, Large domiciliary care)

This person, like others, reported lack of consistency in the time when care staff would arrive, which she found particularly difficult because her husband – a diabetic – had to have his insulin and breakfast at a consistent time.

This exchange, from a different respondent, confirms a pattern of erratic and unsatisfactory care:

> *Interviewer:* How long did you use the [large domiciliary care provider] for?
> *Respondent:* About two months, and believe me it was two months I wouldn't have again.
> *Interviewer:* Was that usually the same person or was that a different person?
> *Respondent:* Oh different girls, but they wasn't carers.
> *Interviewer:* They did the same, so three times a day?
> *Respondent:* Yes, yes but they wasn't here 15 minutes. They came, they made the tea and they went. (Older person 330, Small domiciliary care)

One respondent with a similar experience explains what happened when she complained about the poor service:

> "'Well, we don't get that many ...' – this was the social worker – 'We don't get that many complaints.' I said, 'Well no of course you don't, because people are just grateful for what they get'." (Older person 331, Small domiciliary care)

This is an important point: older people are known to be reluctant to complain about poor-quality care services (EHRC, 2011). This is a problem for user satisfaction scores; and was also for the research that we did, if people felt unwilling to tell us their concerns about their care provider. We might expect that to hold true across different organisational size categories, though, and on the whole – as the quotes above illustrate – people using large services were more likely to complain during the interview than were people using smaller services.

Although drawn from a small number of interviews with people with experience of using large agencies, this account substantiates the well-established profile of large care agencies, in which pressures on unit costs can lead to high staff turnover rates (Bolton and Wibberley, 2013; Skills for Care, 2013). A Skills for Care report (2013, p i) identified that the sector average of 24% staff turnover masked large variance between organisations, and highlighted that smaller organisations were less likely than larger ones to have a high staff turnover. The report also identified higher than average turnover in micro-organisations with under 10 staff, but suggested that this was likely to be because of the large-percentage impact of one or two people leaving (Skills for Care, 2013, p 17).

Accessibility

A third aspect of micro-enterprises that people using the service valued was the high level of *accessibility* of managers. People using micro-enterprises appreciated the close contact they had with the people running the organisation (indeed, for the sole traders in the sample there was no management structure at all).

> "I feel happier knowing that they're a smaller company, somehow, and the lady in charge is the person you can speak to and everything." (Older person 328, Small domiciliary care)

> "There's room out there for a few more like [the provider], they are more personalised and friendly, they know his needs. Because they are small you see everyone, they come to the house, it's not just someone stuck behind a desk. They'll run things past us, let us know what's going on. They give us plenty of feedback, make sure we're satisfied with what they are up to." (Carer 121, Micro day service)

For this family, this level of communication was in marked contrast to the experience they had had with a larger support provider:

> "I've never been let down … Which used to happen with [the larger provider]. I mean, we'd get a phone call off my brother, 'Nobody's called. I've got no tea'." (Carer 121, Micro day service)

Micro-enterprises saw their availability as a key part of their offer:

> "[T]here's also that they can get hold of me 24 hours a day 7 days a week, unless I'm on holiday or something, whereas sort of social services and council services seem to shut down at five o'clock or six o'clock, so if they want to go to the cinema at eight o'clock at night it's generally they can't, they're not very flexible, and they get the certain hours and they get like one o'clock every Wednesday and they might not want to do something at one o'clock every Wednesday, whereas with me they can sort of let me know at the beginning of the week 'can we do this on such a day' and I can sort of schedule myself around them." (Staff 204, Micro day service)

Conclusion

This chapter has focused on the process of care as a way of understanding better the scope for care to lead to particular valued outcomes, and also in recognition of good care as an end in itself. Person-centredness has been analysed as a concept, noting the tendency of much existing work on personalisation to rely either on tautologous definitions or personal testimonies that don't unpack different aspects of person-centredness. We have drawn on the data to extract four ways in which person-centredness is enacted: as flexibility; as anticipation of needs; as acting more like a friend or family member; and as choice and control. The first three of these aspects were found to be more likely in micro and small-scale organisations rather than in larger ones. In relation to choice and control, it has been argued that choice of options can be offered by large day centres, and that this is something that people value. Control is a rather different concept, and in the interviews this was most clearly explained in terms of people feeling a lack of control in the home care services from large providers. Operating at a small scale can provide more personalised support, in ways that seem to be particularly valued in people's homes. In explaining the findings that micro-enterprises tended to be more personalised than larger providers we have drawn on three explanations centred on the autonomy, flexibility and accessibility of these organisations. The next chapter looks at a second aspect of the process of care: the extent to which the services offered are innovative.

EIGHT

Micro innovation: what, how and who?

There has been great optimism about the scope of micro-enterprises to deliver innovative care (Putting People First, 2007; DH and NAAPS, 2009; DH, 2010). This stems from the suggestion that the informal and often fluid nature of micro-enterprises mean that they can be more creative and flexible than large providers and less bounded by traditional service demarcations (Lockwood, 2013). This chapter considers how far those claims are credible. It focuses on innovation as the second of our two measures of process, which locates it in the black box between inputs and outcomes. The main data source for this chapter is the interviews with people running micro-enterprises, although we do also draw on interview data from people who use services where they drew attention to innovative aspects of care.

Measuring and defining innovation is a complex process and many different definitions of innovation have been put forward by academics and practitioners, as discussed in Chapter Two. As with personalisation, the process of undertaking the research allowed us to develop a better understanding of the types of innovation that were apparent in care and support. After a first phase of coding in which we categorised all aspects of innovative practice together, we proceeded abductively to reanalyse the innovation data using the innovative and policy literature to help refine innovation categories. In the next phase of coding, we separated out *what* innovations, *how* innovations and *who* innovations. The first two of these categories came from existing innovation literature, whereas the third emerged from the claims about micro-enterprises that are made in the policy literature, discussed further below.

Types of innovation

Definitions of innovation often stem from the business literature and are particularly focused around 'product' innovation, that is, the production of new types of goods or services (Williams, 2010). Within a healthcare setting, product innovations tend to be associated with a new technology or treatment (Pearson and Rawlins, 2005). Product innovations are also central to generating incremental revenues for many organisations, including in healthcare (Omachonu and Einspruch, 2010). Product innovations therefore refer to what is produced or delivered, and here we refer to it as a *what* innovation.

An alternative form is 'process' innovation, which refers to how a service is delivered and normally includes the introduction of new organisational structures or improved organisational practices (Edquist et al, 2001). Referred to by Williams (2010, pp 146–7) as a *how* innovation, this can relate to changes to organisational processes that may affect communication and relationships inside and outside the organisation. Within healthcare, *how* innovations are often concerned with safeguarding and improving quality (Omachonu and Einspruch, 2010). Within social care, *how* innovations could be linked to the personalisation agenda, both as an external policy driving market changes and also within internal organisational processes when services strive to deliver care in a more person-centred way.

Innovation can also arise as a result of involving citizens and service users in different ways. We refer to this as a *who* innovation. While *who* innovation is not a category used in the academic literature on innovation, it is clear from the policy literature that user involvement and support for potentially marginalised communities is part of the perceived added value of micro-enterprises (DH and NAAPS, 2009; Community Catalysts, 2014). This supports a shift towards co-production, in recognition that the production of a service is difficult without the active participation of those receiving the service (Brandsen and Pestoff, 2006). Co-production can drive innovation by overturning the conventional passive relationship between the consumers of services and those who serve them (Needham and Carr, 2009). Organisations can also undertake *who* innovation in relation to who uses the service, by targeting their service at 'non-traditional' groups of people and responding to their needs in ways that mainstream services have not always done well (Needham and Carr, 2015).

Box 8.1 sets the three types of innovation in a care context. We now turn to consider how these three types of innovation are demonstrated within micro-enterprises and larger social care providers.

Box 8.1: Care sector innovation

Care providers can potentially display three types of innovation

What innovations – creative and alternative types of care

How innovations – more rapid, flexible and responsive care

Who innovations – inclusive of potentially marginalised groups in care service design or delivery

What innovations

Product or *what* innovations refer to which goods are produced or, in service settings, which services are delivered (Edquist et al, 2001; Walker, 2014). Within social care, *what* innovations can be defined as services that deviate from traditional residential, domiciliary and day service models of care. *What* innovations can include services that span the boundaries of these models, for example by using sport, creative activities, multi-sensory activities, work integration or community engagement (DH and NAAPS, 2009). *What* innovations were seen by the micro-enterprises themselves (and the coordinators who supported them in each locality) as their distinctive contribution.

> "So smaller organisations and micro services tend to think more innovatively and outside the box and think of different ways of delivering services. And a lot of the micros ... they don't always perceive themselves as social care organisations so, you know, we've got people like photographers ... we've got somebody who does fishing, we've got somebody does beauty therapy, bread therapy, we've got lots of different services but it's all linked to social care, but it's sort of looking at the holistic approach and not just the traditional methods." (Micro-enterprise co-ordinator 102)

However, as discussed in Chapter Five, many of these more innovative organisations were not included in our sample, either because they had only recently begun trading or because they lacked sufficient regular users for us to be able to assess their quality. We acknowledge that the inclusion only of more established organisations is a limitation on the insights we can offer in relation to innovation.

Of the different types of care service in our sample, we found that one-to-one support services were the most likely to offer *what* innovations, as they took more flexible and individualised approaches to support. People with learning disabilities were more exposed to *what* innovations than were older people, as they engaged in more activities outside the home. These included opportunities for community integration, with activities explicitly aimed at enabling social inclusion and confidence building. In the following example, a micro-enterprise had supported someone with learning disabilities to access the local golf club, and in doing so helped the club to make itself more accessible to a diverse community of people.

> "There's always a certain type of people that go to a golf club but [the club manager] wants to break down that barrier so that everybody can go to golf clubs because everyone's always a bit like oh, sometimes they're really posh and it costs like £2,000 to become a member ... But [he] wants to break down that barrier and he wants everybody to be able to access the facilities there and he wants especially people with learning disabilities." (Staff 107, Micro one-to-one support)

For the older people we interviewed, *what* innovations were less evident, as care most frequently revolved around personal care or other support in the home, including cleaning. However, some services that were classed as domiciliary or one-to-one support in the home did offer support in addition to personal care or cleaning. This included providing opportunities for older people to socially engage, such as trips out to local cafes and stately homes. Box 8.2 sets out an example of a micro-enterprise offering a *what* innovation.

Box 8.2: Demonstrating *what* innovation

Creative Vision is a micro-enterprise that was established to deliver creative activities to older people in nursing and residential homes. Activities in the nursing homes are varied depending on the needs of the people being supported and include reminiscence, sensory workshops and arts and crafts sessions. The organisation also provides opportunities for retired, socially isolated people to volunteer in nursing homes, for example as a singer. As the owner explains:

> "So it's about using activity and using not necessarily creative activity but creative ideas, you know, so often people think of creative then think oh it's card making, but it's about creative thinking ... I see this as a value-led organisation and that's at its core I think, you know, if it just becomes another provider then it's going to lose the whole point of what it was doing or just sit alongside them rather than offering anything new or different." (Staff 303, Micro day service)

In relation to size of provider, it was micro-enterprises that were more likely than large providers to offer one-to-one support and to allow staff the flexibility to be varied in the support given, as discussed in the last chapter. We therefore found a range of *what* innovations within micro-enterprises. However, these were not unique to micro-providers, as our interviews also provided evidence of *what* innovation within larger care services. As indicated in Chapter Two, previous literature on innovation indicates that larger organisations often have more resources, including money and staff, allowing greater investment, particularly in *what* innovations, than smaller organisations (Camison Zornoza et al, 2004; Damanpour et al, 2009). This was evident in some of the larger case study organisations that were found to invest resources in innovative activities. This was displayed in one medium-sized local authority day centre where the manager talked about the future of the centre as a hub for a range of care services, including micro-enterprises.

> "I can see us becoming a little market place almost in a way so that ... the council building if you like becomes the hub and within that you've got like little providers. I mean we also knit with some of the other micro-providers to currently provide some of the activities, so we're slowly becoming like a little market place." (Staff 111, Medium day service)

In another locality, the closure of several local authority day centres had led to the establishment of one large centre providing integrated services for older people, people with learning disabilities and people with physical difficulties. Although driven by the need for more cost-effective and efficient care services, this is arguably a *what* innovation in day centre provision, as the new, integrated model of care was considerably different to the previous model, where people with different social care needs were separated into different day centres. Despite uncertainty from staff and centre attendees at the outset, the new, integrated centre is perceived to have led to enhanced social integration by breaking down the barriers between older people and people with learning disabilities. One staff member reflected:

> "When I thought God, this is working, I was in the coffee bar and I was sitting having my lunch and I just looked and all the chairs had been moved around and people had pulled them together to sit together. And there was the guy with early onset dementia, he had his iPad out and he was showing some photographs of his motorbike and there was a couple of older people that were saying 'I used to have this

motorbike when I was young' or 'I remember my husband and I ...' and there was a couple of people with learning disabilities saying 'I'd love to ride on a motorbike' and they were all talking, it was an actual conversation that was criss-crossing and going all over and I thought this is working, this is how it should be." (Staff 307, Large day service)

As discussed in the previous chapter, larger day centres were also often able to provide a greater range of activities than were small day centres.

It is also important to acknowledge that *what* innovations may be easier to introduce when people have low to moderate levels of need, and may become less prevalent as levels of frailty increase. The flexible one-to-one support model offered by several of the micro-enterprises, in which people could undertake a range of activities outside the home on an ad hoc basis, may become less appropriate as people's levels of frailty increase. Indeed, some carers felt that micro-enterprises could not cope as well as larger providers with the intensity of supporting someone whose needs were more complex:

"I think they do an excellent job of supporting [someone at the early stages of dementia], but I think as the needs get higher and it's perhaps becoming more complicated and you probably need staff who need specific dementia care training, maybe [the micro] are not quite at that level yet." (Carer 108, Micro domiciliary care)

It may also be about the time demands of someone with 24-hour care needs, or who requires emergency cover. The same person reflected, "I think that's possibly the negative side of a micro, is that they may not necessarily have the expanse of staff to be able to really pull on in an emergency ..."

Some carers were happy to source the emergency and night-time cover from other agencies and to continue to use the micro-enterprise during the day. For others, the complexity of managing relationships with lots of different providers was difficult and they preferred to respond to growing needs by commissioning support from a larger organisation that could provide everything. Two of the people we interviewed were about to end their contract with micro-enterprises that had provided care for several years, in both cases because their family member's dementia had advanced to such a level that the micro support was no longer adequate. One person was going into residential care. The other was to be supported in her home by a larger agency. In this latter case, her daughter told us:

> "I'm actually shopping around [for an alternative to the micro]. I had a chat to this particular [larger] company and I said 'well, you know, what is your back-up', because I think that's my issue at the moment is what is really the back-up. And they've got three permanent people on call, so they employ somebody who's on call all the time, then they have the manager and the assistant manager who are also on call and then they also put in cover for when one of them is on holiday. So there's three people permanently on call. And they don't have that at [the micro]." (Carer 108, Micro domiciliary care)

This discussion suggests that micro-enterprises are likely to be most effective when supporting people at a lower level of need, where more creative and community-based *what* innovations may be easier to introduce.

How innovations

Although micro-enterprises did give some examples of *what* innovations as indicated above, the limitations of the sample meant that it was difficult to fully appraise the claims that are made for micro-enterprises in relation to redefining what is meant by 'care'. In relation to *how* innovations it was easier to undertake comparisons between the different-sized organisations in our sample. *How* innovations relate to the process through which a service is delivered (Williams, 2010).

The difference between *what* and *how* innovations is perhaps demonstrated most clearly in relation to frail older people in what Gilleard and Higgs (2010) call the 'fourth age' of life. Higgs and Gilleard (2015) write about the fourth age as a level of frailty that people must reach in order to receive state-funded care services and that contrasts with the third age of active retirees, heavily invested in consumption and leisure activities. They argue: 'The frailed individual is caught in a system of care that is doled out, rationed and increasingly driven by a rhetoric of choice within a social reality made up of constraint and dependency' (Higgs and Gilleard, 2015, p 77). A number of authors have argued that the innovative approaches to care promised by the personalisation narrative are not realisable for these frail older people (Lloyd, 2014). Similarly, Age UK has pointed out that care services for older people stand in contrast to services for younger disabled people, for whom 'personal budgets can be relatively large and there is a real focus on "living life" when planning support, whereas personal budgets for older people are often considered to be purely about personal care and maintenance and, as a result, tend to be much smaller' (Age UK, 2013, p 71).

Our research suggests that even in cases where the scope for *what* innovations may be very limited – for example, if resource and mobility constraints make it difficult for people to leave the home – there is still scope for *how* innovation in relation to person-centred care. The micro and small organisations in our sample appeared better able than the larger organisations to be flexible and spontaneous in the care provided – a form of enacted personalisation, discussed in the previous chapter. Flexibility could include having a drink or meal with the older person in their home, as this micro-enterprise coordinator told us:

> "We have got a lot of traditional [micro-enterprise] services, so we've got a lot of people who do, sort of, home help type of services, you know, the shopping, the cleaning, meal preparation, but it's their approach to it [that's different], so for example one of the micros that I work with, they'll do meal preparation but they'll sit down and have the meal with that person and interact with that person." (Micro-enterprise coordinator 101)

Micro-enterprises in some cases were willing to provide additional unpaid support to their service users, including respite and support to carers.

> "[The service user] who comes today, her daughter's been away for the first time in years … [I went] round and put her support stockings on for her in the morning before she came in [to the day centre] because otherwise, she don't get carers, her daughter wouldn't be able to go away. And you know, maybe I shouldn't do that but I just see it that if that gives that little bit of respite, you know that's helping the Council because otherwise [the service user] would have to go into a home or her daughter wouldn't have got away and then where would her daughter be? Her daughter would get to crisis point." (Staff 302, Micro day service)

We did not hear examples of these kinds of *how* innovations – linked closely to enacted personalisation – outside of the micro-enterprises and small providers in our study.

Who innovations

The data analysis also identified an additional way in which care services can be innovative, which we term *who* innovations and relates to the people with which the organisations engage. Services that are run by or co-produced with people who use services facilitated the empowerment of potentially marginalised people by integrating the service itself more effectively into the local community. Enabling people with care needs to establish and run care services can arguably unlock innovation by allowing the development of more responsive services tailored to the needs of those who use them (DH and NAAPS, 2009).

Two forms of *who* innovation were encountered: the first relates to the people running the organisations and the second relates to the extent to which the organisation engaged with and supported a diverse range of people.

The two user-led organisations in our sample were run by people with learning disabilities and were micro-enterprises (see Box 8.3 for an example).

Box 8.3: Involving people with learning disabilities in running a micro-enterprise

The A Team is a football club set up and run by someone with learning disabilities. The founder of the club saw the need for the service because of his own negative experiences of other football groups that excluded people with disabilities. He felt a more relaxed approach was needed to allow people with disabilities to fully enjoy their active time, as he explains:

> "I went in as a footballer [to another local football club], tried it for myself and the coach we didn't get on, me and him, and basically I tried to look elsewhere to open up something else that was for me. In our club I'm laid back enough to let them free, you know do what they want, up to a certain extent. In other clubs people told players what to do, really be very, very more or less vicious to them and I'm not like that." (Person with learning disability 202, Micro day service)

Other micro-enterprises were not user led but did provide employment to service users.

> "Part of the reason for setting up my own company was to actually employ people who had different and unique needs to a) get work experience b) to set up a micro-enterprise, a co-operative. I'm not aware that [the local area] has a co-operative micro-enterprise with people who experience different needs. And I wanted to really empower people from the beginning." (Staff 206, Micro day service)

In a third model, people using the service were involved in designing the support and activities provided.

> "We offer such a variety of activities. It's user led, so they tell us what they want to do and then we have to engineer a programme round that ... One of the issues we found when we first started was that all our members were vocal, but they'd got a lot of friends who weren't. So they wanted to continue learning Makaton so that they could communicate with their friends that they'd got elsewhere that weren't. So that was fantastic." (Staff 108, Micro day service)

Co-production was also evident in some of the larger care and support services. A large day centre for people with learning disabilities worked hard at user engagement, and hosted a user-led information and advocacy service within it. A national charity that provides accommodation for people with learning disabilities in one of our localities also articulated a strong commitment to building mutual support based on the expertise and skills of the people who use the service. All of these examples of types of engagement – micro and larger – were taken from services for people with learning disabilities; in our sample, we didn't find any examples of older people being involved in service management or design. While this may be reflective of the limits of our sample, it does accord with broader concerns about the extent to which younger people's services emphasise 'living life', whereas older people's services are limited to physical maintenance (Age UK, 2013).

The second type of *who* innovation related to the ability of providers to engage with a diverse range of people who use services, including BME communities and other 'seldom heard' groups such as LGBT communities. We included three organisations in the sample that were primarily oriented to people from BME communities, but did not find any LGBT-oriented organisations with an established set of people using the services.

Staff from the micro-enterprises supporting people from BME communities spoke about how they felt that they provided a unique offer for people from that community. This included providing care and support services for South Asian women, a potentially marginalised group who are known to be wary of seeking help from statutory services (Kotecha, 2009; Edge, 2011). One micro-enterprise was able to engage with South Asian women who were unable to access any other help and support as a result of service closures.

> "Because it reaches out to women from the South Asian culture because a service has closed, there was nothing there for these women and it's all around like having female support basically and being with other females. So it's sort of – I suppose it's become our unique selling point really."
> (Staff 203, Micro day service)

Previous research has identified that BME and other 'seldom heard' communities often feel marginalised from mainstream care and support services, which may not cater for cultural and language differences. Furthermore, traditional care services can discriminate against BME and other 'seldom heard' groups, especially large, mainstream or generalist providers (Sin, 2006; Needham and Carr, 2015). Our research found examples of care being self-organised and provided on an informal basis, as explained by someone from a small support organisation within the Chinese community.

> "They tried to put [older person with care needs] into a nursing home which is only English spoken and if, you know, English people that run that and he didn't like to go in ... He couldn't understand anything at all. So I went in to help ... I looked after him for eight hours per day."
> (Staff 309, Small one-to-one support)

Some of the micro-enterprises were able to bridge the boundaries between BME communities and statutory care providers, not only by breaking down language barriers but also through the generation of trust and shared understanding (Box 8.4).

Box 8.4: Brokering relationships with marginalised communities

Abdul left social work to set up Active Support, an agency supporting young people with autism and learning disabilities. Most of the people supported are from South Asian communities. As well as offering day activities, the organisation provides one-to-one support for people with complex needs. In one example, Abdul and his staff have been working with a family for several months to address the continence issues of the adult son, who has autism. A community nurse, who has been supporting the family over a longer period, spoke to us when we visited the family home, explaining that it was not until the involvement of Abdul that progress had been made. While this example is not from a formal research interview, we include it here because of the perspective it gives on how the family have been supported by the micro-enterprise:

> "The fact that [Abdul] knows the family and can speak the language has really helped to make progress on the continence issue. I had been to visit the family a couple of times with an independent interpreter but I wasn't really able to establish a relationship with them that way. With [Abdul], they know and trust him and that makes a big difference. And also with the client himself, if he sees me and knows that I come with [Abdul] then he thinks I'm OK, he doesn't mind me being there." (Community nurse)

While efforts have been made by statutory bodies to improve services especially for BME communities, Bowes and Dar (2000) argue that problems of ethnocentricity and accessibility remain. In a review of existing literature on access to care services among potentially marginalised communities, Needham and Carr (2015) put forward a number of reasons for non-engagement with or disengagement from mainstream care and support by BME communities, LGBT people, refugees and asylum seekers. These include: homogenisation and diversity blindness, as service providers can lack cultural sensitivity by homogenising or over-generalising racial or ethnic characteristics; language and communication, which is seen as a 'source of enduring difficulty' for people from BME communities who are not fluent in English; assumptions about the role of friends and family as carers among some BME communities; cultural issues of stigma around using care services, especially mental health services. The review concluded that 'it is apparent that people and communities who have found traditional, mainstream services inappropriate or problematic to engage with, can be instrumental in finding appropriate solutions themselves', through small, community-based organisations (Needham and Carr, 2015, p 8).

Conclusion

The relationship between organisation size and innovation has been debated by academics and policy makers for many decades. This chapter has identified the different types of innovation that are displayed within the specific context of care; we refer to these as *what, how* and *who* innovations. In terms of *what* innovations, some micro-enterprises within our sample are delivering services that deviate from the traditional residential, domiciliary and day models of care through the provision of flexible 'one-to-one support'. While micro-enterprises were offering more flexible services, larger organisations were also offering a broad range of services and, in day provision especially, larger services were found to offer more choice to service users.

Many of the micro-enterprises, especially those supporting people with learning disabilities, tended to have an active relationship with service users, supporting the empowerment of service users as 'active citizens' to run or co-produce services, which we class here as *who* innovation. Again, we encountered examples of large organisations also working co-productively to involve people who use services in designing and managing those services. The distinctive contribution of micro-enterprises seemed to be more specifically in targeting support to potentially marginalised communities, which larger services are known to have a poor record of including. Our sample allowed us to explore this only in relation to BME communities, although existing literature does highlight that small community organisations have emerged to offer targeted support for groups such as LGBT people and traveller communities (Needham and Carr, 2015).

While it tends to be the *what* and *who* innovations within micro-enterprises that are most widely reported (Daly, 2013; DH and NAAPS, 2009), it may be the *how* innovations that are most important when it comes to the context of social care for older people. For people receiving personal care in the home, the scope for micro providers to take a more flexible approach gives them an advantage over large care providers.

Taken together, Chapters Six to Eight have presented the case for micro-enterprises having the potential to offer care that achieves valued and cost-effective outcomes, offers certain kinds of innovation and is person-centred. The next two chapters discuss these findings, highlighting the aspects of micro-enterprises that appear to make them perform better than larger care providers. They also consider some of the limitations of micro–enterprises, for example in relation to organisational sustainability and local authority support, which create limits to their effectiveness.

NINE

How micro-enterprise performs

This chapter focuses on explaining why micro-enterprises are able to perform well on the four measures we used in the study. We begin by revisiting the hypotheses set out in Chapter Three, and consider them in the context of the evidence presented in Chapters Six, Seven and Eight. We then focus on explaining why it is that micro-enterprises perform better than larger organisations. Part of this relates to organisational structures, with very small organisations being more flexible and informal than larger ones. However, we go on to argue that structural explanations cannot fully explain our findings. There are aspects of smallness that are performative in the sense of being 'generative of practices that produce particular forms of performance' (Skelcher, 2008, p 40). Micro-enterprise is performed in the claims that are made for it as an identity and ethos that differentiates it from larger providers.

Returning to the hypotheses

The first hypothesis stated that micro-enterprises were better at achieving valued outcomes than larger providers, and the ASCOT data presented in Chapter Six indicated that this was the case on both of the dimensions tested (spending time on things I value and enjoy; having choice and control in my daily life). Only the first of these was statistically significant, and the small numbers in our study are more broadly a limit on the generalisability of these findings. The qualitative data also highlighted the limitations of quantitative outcomes-based measures, given that many of the older people in our sample wanted to talk about the process of care rather than articulate an outcome.

In relation to the second hypothesis – value for money – we set pricing data from the different-sized organisations alongside the outcomes data to argue that micro-enterprises do constitute good value for money. However, in Chapter Six we also provided a broader discussion of the contextual factors shaping care pricing, and the extent to which micro-enterprises are limited to serving largely self-funders and people with direct payments. For local authority-commissioned care services, large providers do remain the cheapest option. We return to the issue of local authority commissioning practices in the next chapter, which focuses on the sustainability of micro care providers.

The third hypothesis focused on personalised care, and in the chapter on enacting personalisation we argued that this was where the benefits of micro-enterprise were most compelling. They were able to provide care that was personalised in a number of different ways (such as anticipating needs and treating people more like a friend or family member). Choice and control were disaggregated in this chapter, since some of the larger organisations seemed to offer a wider range of choices, but it was in relation to the micro-organisations that people felt more control. Continuity of staff, the ability of staff to be flexible in the support provided and accessibility of managers were key aspects of the enactment of person-centred care.

The fourth hypothesis was that micro-enterprises were more innovative than larger providers. Our research highlighted the need to disaggregate innovation into its different aspects – *what, how* and *who* innovations – noting that for older people's home care, *how* innovation relating to person-centred care was extremely important, while *what* types of innovation were invoked less frequently. While some micro-enterprises were offering completely different types of support service, many were offering services that were recognisable as domiciliary or group support (partly because our sampling approach required that we find organisations that were comparable with larger providers). The main contribution of micro-enterprise was in relation to *how* care was provided and the scope to be more innovative in *who* was involved in designing and delivering support.

Organisational structures

Having summarised the findings in relation to the hypotheses, the next part of the chapter explains why micro-enterprises were able to perform well, as compared to larger providers, drawing attention to two aspects of micro-delivery. The first is that the organisational structures of micro-enterprises facilitated informal modes of working in which flexibility and autonomy were much more attainable than in large organisations. As is known from other research on small firms, there was less focus on adhering to formal procedures and more use of face-to-face and informal communication (Storey, 1994; Edwards et al, 2004). Some of the micro-enterprises were sole traders, others operated with staff but the founders were still highly involved in the planning of care, providing some of the care services themselves. Staff could vary the service on the day, make decisions about what to do and be available to clients and families because there were few clients and an almost horizontal staffing structure.

These findings give support to the argument set out in Chapter Two, that the inherent advantage of small organisations when it comes to innovation is their flexibility and the ability to accept and implement changes more readily than do larger organisations (Damanpour, 1996). The owner of one micro-enterprise gave her perspective on the different working practices of large and small care services:

> "You know you're not going through a load of red tape, you're not saying 'I'll have to ask my manager', we just crack on with it you know. I mean we follow all Health and Safety guidelines so we're safe, but there's no constraints on us like there can be in a big organisation. You know, 'you can't do this because of this or you're short staffed' or whatever, we just crack on." (Staff 204, Micro day service)

People running micro-enterprises see themselves as being able to try out new ideas and develop services that are more flexible, responsive and centred on the needs of the people they support.

> "What you do find is in big organisations … you have to go through so many hoops and barriers to do everything and you can't make any decisions and get things done right away. Whereas, if you're a micro-enterprise you can respond every minute to what the needs are." (Staff 108, Micro day service)

This ability to try out new ideas and 'crack on' could be seen as a weakness in the regulation of the micro-enterprise sector. Micro-enterprises are not registered with the CQC if they are not providing regulated services such as domiciliary or residential care. However, we were not aware during the research of any unsafe practice, nor were any safety concerns raised with us by the people using the services (micro or larger). We did find that several micro-providers said they wanted to get CQC registration (which would allow them to offer a wider range of services) but felt that the process of doing so was too lengthy and costly for them. The need to ensure that regulation is proportional for very small organisations is a theme returned to in Chapter Ten.

Managers in the large organisations that we spoke to operated in more complex and formally organised structures. The large domiciliary care agency we included in the study had 135 staff and provided care services to 350 people, which necessitated several layers of management and the use of technology to manage rostering. Indeed, the owner of the organisation framed its distinctive 'offer' in terms of the technology it used:

> "We have call monitoring/alarms so if someone hasn't visited we know about it, and we will get someone there within 45 minutes, even if is 11pm at night ... We have electronic rostering, and not text messaging." (Staff 113, Large domiciliary care)

In contrast, in the micro-enterprises and small care providers that we interviewed the distinctive offer was framed more in terms of interpersonal relationships ("We say to the client, 'What do you want? What time do you want to go to bed?' And if they say 8:30, or 8:15, or 9:15, that's what we do" (Staff 103, Micro domiciliary care)).

It is important to note that the one large domiciliary provider that we included did not display some of the features that have been criticised in other large care providers: it was a local, family-owned firm, rather than being a large, national chain financed through private equity funding (Land and Himmelweit, 2010). The company paid its staff for travel time and cited a lower staff turnover rate than the sector average. It was also willing to take part in the research, and was the only large domiciliary provider that agreed to do so. However, even with these factors borne in mind it was clear from interviews with people who received care services from this organisation that its working practices did not deliver the personalised and consistent care that the people using the service wanted: care visits were short and there was a lack of staff continuity. The extent to which this reflects the parameters that the commissioning local authorities placed on the organisation is discussed in the next chapter.

Micro as identity

Organisational simplicity, then, is one of the factors that explains why micro-enterprises are more person centred and innovative than larger providers. A second explanatory factor is related more strongly to identity rather than the formal aspects of organisational design, and focuses on the scale of organisations. This is a comparative measure of how they are located in a distribution of different size providers of care. Postma draws attention to the difference between size and scale:

scales can be defined as *socially constructed hierarchically nested spaces*. In other words: a scale is a space that is demarcated by social action, hierarchically related to other spaces (e.g. small versus large, micro versus macro, global versus local) and endowed with meaning (e.g. the community, the nation state, the European Union). This distinguishes scale from size: size is an absolute measure of a phenomenon, while scale denotes the relation between different phenomena. (Postma, 2015, p 92)

Postma's work usefully draws attention to the relative perspectives that are captured in the notion of scale. In his research on Dutch healthcare providers, he explores the 'scalar narratives' through which 'people endow scales with meaning and frame them as real and legitimate sites of social action and the execution of power' (Postma, 2015, p 93). In researching 'the rhetorical use of scalar practices' in Dutch news stories about health he found accounts of senior executives being said to be 'miles away' in large organisations, whereas the small-scale was associated with 'idealistic notions of personal attention, warmth, empathy and benevolent professionals' (Postma, 2015, p 105).

This analysis highlights the performative aspect of the micro label, beyond the formal organisational attribute of staff numbers. Performativity is a term that covers a range of theoretical insights, associated with the work of Lyotard (1984), Butler (1993) and Callon (2007), among others. It has been introduced into public policy and institutional contexts by a range of scholars including Hajer (2006), Peck and Dickinson (2009) and Dickinson (2014). Hajer's work draws attention to the ways in which 'actors enact performances in which the *contextualized interaction* itself produces social realities such as understandings of the problem at hand, knowledge, new power relations, and trust' (Hajer 2006, p 49, emphasis in original).

That micro-enterprise held these generative properties was evident in our interviews. The people we were interviewing were primed to talk about themselves as 'micros'. As one interviewee put it:

> "I'm very micro at the moment in that it's just me and that's the difficult part because of resources, you know …. For me as a micro-enterprise I would rather be self-sufficient, sustainable." (Staff 108, Micro day service)

Their identity had been established partly through the work of the local micro-enterprise coordinators in helping these organisations to get started and including them in a local micro-provider forum, and partly through defining themselves in opposition to the larger providers. It was also notable that some of the larger organisations were aware of local micro-enterprise activity and sought to talk about their own work in those terms, affirming the purchase of the 'micro' label as a benchmark of a personalised service. An interviewee running a small franchise of a large national care chain said:

> "Our ethos is very much like the micro providers … I know every single one of our clients, I interviewed every single one of our care givers and know every single one of our care givers." (Staff 112, Small domiciliary care)

For the micro-enterprises themselves the notion of scale was important in the ways that Postma (2015) suggests: large was portrayed as dystopian, as compared to the intimacy of smaller provision. For some people this was based on what they had heard from the people for whom they were providing care and support:

> "The [local authority] seem to have huge, two or three large companies that just are national and they've started in the village but we've picked up some of theirs because they've (a) not turned up or (b) they're not very good at hygiene. There just seemed to be issues with the size, and I do think that comes with size, from working with a national company. You don't have that much control and we're very personal." (Staff 308, Small domiciliary care)

> "[A large care provider] had really let her down and they weren't flexible, they invoice her every week and they just dropped, say they're not coming, you know, half an hour before which is really difficult for her son to get his head round. You know, he's ready to go out and then suddenly …" (Staff 9, Micro one-to-one support)

For others it reflected experiences they had had during their careers in observing how large institutions operated.

> "The big hospital in Leeds, people with learning disabilities, one of the big institutions and I can remember going in some of the workshops and thinking never, ever, ever. It was just rows and rows and rows of people taking plastic

bits off skateboard wheels ... [I was] just thinking this is dreadful." (Staff 205, Micro day service)

"Smaller is better, that's my opinion because I've been to care homes where, you know, obviously they've got a big capacity there but again the chairs around the edge of the room and you've got a television blasting out and you've got a radio at the same time blasting out and staff are very busy and they're all just sitting there lost." (Staff 305, Large day service)

Another person recounted his own personal experience of working for a large care provider:

"I had been working for a very, very large organisation and as a kind of regional manager type thing [with] people who had experience of very complex needs, especially around learning disability, autism ... and for me the whole thrust was quality work. But the thrust of the organisation began to morph into volume and it felt a bit like battery farming people and I was told basically, well, I was encouraged ... go out there and market, market, market and I can market, market, market, but I'm a kind of person who has very personal reasons for doing quality, quality, quality that's why I chose to go into the profession. So we agreed to differ and I then set up my own company." (Staff 206, Micro day service)

The investment in being micro that we found in the people who had set up the micro-enterprises may in part be a manifestation of entrepreneurial attitudes more generally. As Fenwick (2002) argues, developing a new enterprise can be bound up with self-development, with work becoming a place to carve out a space to flourish not only economically, but also socially, intellectually and emotionally. Furthermore, the balancing of work and personal/family life can transgress discourses of profitability, productivity and success, especially for women starting up their own business (Fenwick, 2002). Eighty per cent of the micro-enterprise founders in our sample were women, reflective of care as a traditionally female occupation (Ungerson, 1983). In addition, research on spin-outs in health and other sectors has also indicated that desires for personal profitability are less likely to motivate staff than opportunities to improve work satisfaction and improve outcomes and access to services for patients (Hall et al, 2012b; Hazenberg and Hall, 2014).

In relation to care services, there may be a further, more immediately personal motivation. While the quotes above drew attention to people who were motivated to set up micro-enterprises because of their poor experiences of working in large providers, several of the micro-enterprises had been created by people because of the bad experiences of care that they had witnessed within their own families. In these cases the motivation to develop a micro care service stemmed from frustrations as a parent. This interviewee, who has a son with an autism diagnosis, explains:

> "if I'm honest – it sounds arrogant – as a parent, as a purchaser of services and also purchasing services for two elderly relatives (my mother-in-law and my own father), I thought, 'I can do better than this. I can certainly do it different and more person-centred.' And, you know, we've had courses through [the council] telling us what personalisation is; I've been doing it for 20-odd years, before the word was invented." (Staff 103, Micro domiciliary care)

The experience of being a parent negotiating services afforded a particular insight into where the gaps are in mainstream provision. A different micro-enterprise, also run by the parent of a child with autism, demonstrates a whole-family approach that has helped to provide stability for one service user with autism:

> "One of the people [I support] has had 21 placements in the first 16 years of his life until I became involved and then that was it, sorted. Again, lots of time and listening to different parties went into that as well as some specialist knowledge." (Staff 206, micro day service)

The notion of large-scale as a symbolic representation of depersonalised and poor-quality care was also evident in the interviews with people who used services and with carers. For some this came from direct experience. One family carer described how she felt she was listened to when using a micro day service, in a way she had not been when approaching a larger provider.

> "Yeah, because they listen and that's the main thing ... you go to other places and it just goes in – what you say 'oh

well you do this because she's such and such' and it just goes in one ear and out the other. But they actually listen and they take note and they do as much as they can to help her." (Carer 209, Micro day service)

A person with learning disabilities who purchased services from a micro-enterprise talked about how apprehensive they would be towards a larger service, based on a previous experience:

"I went to a Day Centre years ago and there were loads there, I wouldn't like it. If it was small though I wouldn't mind it, but I think it's too much when it's loads of people sometimes." (Person with learning disabilities 224, Micro day service)

For many interviewees, large-scale care was a spectre, a feared imaginary even when they had no direct or recent experience of it themselves. Even someone who was currently supported by a medium-sized organisation talked about what she felt would be lost if she was to get care from a large company instead:

"All these little things I think would disappear, various things. She'll say 'I know you like fresh air. I know you like your windows open. Shall I open that one up there', sort of thing. But all these little, very unimportant details to other people, I think you lose in a bigger organisation 'cos they don't know you intimately." (Older person 322, Medium one-to-one support)

The notion of large-scale care as a sort of imagined bogeyman was also evident in this interview, from someone with no personal experience of a large provider:

"I've heard – you know how you hear these little bits from people who come – I've heard people who have a bigger organisation and somebody coming in four times a day and that sort of thing." (Older person 316, Small domiciliary care)

The tone used by the interviewee made clear that she saw this 'four times a day' model of care as undesirable.

What is clear in the quotes above is the emotional investment in smallness as opposed to largeness. In these depictions of large-scale care provision – the language of 'rows and rows of people', of 'battery farming' – the interviewees (people running micro-enterprises and people using care services) associate large scale with the dystopian and depersonalised.

Staying micro

One of the issues discussed in Chapter Two was the difficulty of working with size as a variable because of its dynamic nature, with organisations fluctuating over time. It was suggested from the academic and policy literature that micro care providers might prefer to stay small, rather than locate themselves on a trajectory towards growth. This claim puts them out of kilter with the mainstream of emerging businesses in which growth is assumed to be a shared aspiration (Mueller, 1972; Ram and Trehan, 2010, p 420; Dellot, 2014).

Given the negative associations that many of the micro-enterprises held towards large-scale care provision, it is unsurprising that many of them were wary of organisational growth. Nonetheless, almost all of the micro-enterprises interviewed for the research planned to grow slightly bigger. This was as true for the sole trader as it was for the multi-staff micro pushing at the limits of the micro category. The pressure for growth was coming either from their own need to break even financially, or from demand by clients for additional services. One micro-enterprise, providing group and one-to-one support for people with learning disabilities, described a desire to grow but a concern that he was pigeon-holed by social services as an ethnic minority provider, which limited the number of referrals that he got.

> "Referrals are, I think, one of the challenges for me ... The minority community in [the town] isn't that big. The people we work with are mainly Pakistani.... We haven't got that many users. We're getting by, but I could do with more referrals. Now, the challenge for me is to sustain [the business] and for staff, they want more hours' work." (Staff 114, Micro day service)

This difficulty of breaking out of what Ram and Jones (2008) call 'co-ethnic custom' is well established in relation to ethnic-minority small businesses.

However, for all but two micros (which ultimately wanted to franchise their operations), this desire for growth was limited by a self-imposed threshold. For several of them this was shaped by a feeling that at a larger size they would not be able to deliver care according to the same ethos. This threshold was variable between providers. For one it was to have 10 members of staff, for another it was to draw a salary and not keep ploughing his savings into the business to keep it afloat. The following quotes are indicative of the attitudes to growth that we found among the micro-enterprises.

> "I don't think I want to grow. I think I'd probably bring another staff member in but I don't want to grow too much bigger to be honest. I like what we've got. I like the you know, it's personal." (Staff 308, Small domiciliary care)

> "I want to grow, but I don't want to get big if we lose the ethos …If you drew a graph – if there's a line at which – if you could do that in mathematical terms, if you broke through the line that says, 'You're going to lose the ethos', then I wouldn't want to break through that. If it meant that my earnings were 300% increased, I don't want that if we lose that feeling that we have now." (Staff 103, Micro domiciliary care)

As part of maintaining the ethos of a very small organisation, the people running the micro-enterprises wanted to preserve the control that they had over the organisation. Some of them sought flexible and temporary approaches to staffing, which blurred the boundaries between formal and informal support.

> "We have one of the ladies' carers who does a bit of support for us and we were a bit dubious at first but it's been a real positive because she can see what goes on. Then we have a couple of ladies that we've used that we know we can rely on and you know what they're doing." (Staff 303, Micro day service)

Similarly, instead of seeking a solution to this staffing issue based on expansion, one micro care service described adopting a community cohesion approach, with service users' family members working with them to cover absence and leave. This carer, the sister of a service user with complex communication and learning disabilities, explained how she felt part of the micro-enterprise and enjoyed covering staff absences occasionally:

> "I know that [staff member] trusts me enough to say '[The usual care giver] is not in next week can you do two days for me?' 'Yeah, of course I can no problem.' And I love it." (Carer 210, Micro day service)

Again, the organisational boundaries here were fluid and able to absorb informal support to build capacity when required.

Another micro-enterprise owner used her own family members on a casual basis to help increase capacity as needed. For example, the micro-enterprise owner sometimes asked her husband to drive when she was taking the people she supported out for the day. The reliance on ad hoc, informal and often family-based arrangements to increase capacity is known to be a feature of many small firms (Edwards and Ram, 2006). This point also links to the discussion earlier in the book about organisational boundaries as fluid rather than fixed.

Conclusion

In this chapter we have focused on explaining why micro-enterprises performed well on most aspects of our four hypotheses (encompassing improved outcomes, value for money, personalisation and innovative support). It was argued that part of the explanation comes from the organisational simplicity of micro-enterprises, which enables them to be flexible and allows staff and people using services to have easy access to the people running the service (who may also be the person providing the care).

As well as a size category, 'micro' is a scalar identity, which has a performative aspect, generative of particular kinds of care practices. Some of the people who set up micro providers did so out of a core motivation to do care and support differently from larger organisations. As people who had worked in large care providers or used those providers for family members, they had an explicit commitment to work in different ways and to avoid what they saw as the dehumanising nature of much large-scale care work. Many of them identified strongly with the micro label and were reluctant to compromise their distinctive ethos through rapid or substantial organisational growth.

While recognising that organisational flexibility and a scalar account of good care are key strengths of micro-enterprises, it is also important to recognise some of the vulnerabilities that these aspects create for the micro–enterprise model. In the next chapter we consider the business model of micro-enterprise and the relationships that they are able to establish with local authorities. Through this we consider the extent to which they constitute a sustainable model of care provision.

TEN

Sustainability: are micro-enterprises built to last?

Previous chapters have highlighted several aspects of the positive contribution that micro-enterprises can make to care and support services. During the research we also identified factors that facilitated and inhibited how they function. Engaging with changing political and financial contexts and understanding challenges faced by micro providers are central to understanding how they might play an increased role in social care provision in the future. Although the research was designed primarily to evaluate care services and understand their contributions, how micro-sized organisations are situated within the health and social care system and how they relate to other organisations has an impact on their reach and quality of service.

This chapter focuses on four interlinked aspects of micro-enterprises that shape their effectiveness and their likely contribution to future care services. These are: visibility; financial viability; relationship with the local authority; and quality and regulation. These are a combination of factors that are internal and external to the micro-enterprises. They encompass some attributes or structures that the organisations have the power to change and others that lie outside of their control.

The visibility of micro-enterprises

People who coordinated and worked within micro-enterprises, as well as people who used them, frequently commented on the degree to which organisations were well known locally and were visible to potential users. Our analysis suggested a number of positive and more problematic visibility issues faced by micro-enterprises. On one hand, the people running micro-enterprises often had strong links to other local services and typically had experience of working in or using care services for many years. The knowledge and relationships that came from the individuals who started micro-enterprises often put them in a strong position to build a client base and work alongside local partners. However, there was also a strong sense that local authority strategies and processes could limit the progress of micro care providers. This limiting effect was described in a number of ways. Some of the barriers to progress that were identified included a lack of referrals from local authorities, micro-enterprises being left out of provider lists on websites and service users not being fully aware of holding a personal budget or being able to commission their own choice of service provider.

In the following quote a local coordinator elaborates on a broader trend found in this study, that micro-enterprises often play a useful role by utilising their local service knowledge to find new opportunities for service users, making the rest of the system visible.

> "[M]ost of the micros who I've worked with are very much linked with other services ... what I mean by that is if somebody who supported somebody with a learning disability for example but actually they didn't have any space or they didn't have the skills or whatever to support this person, but they knew of an organisation locally that did, they'd tend to more refer people on." (Micro coordinator 301)

This statement encapsulates two findings from the study, drawing attention to the beneficial information-sharing activity of micro care organisations and the scope for micro-enterprises to become part of local networks. The peer support groups for micro-enterprises that existed in two of the three localities were recognised as playing a valued role in providing support, supporting findings from the broader literature about the benefits of 'entrepreneurial networking' (Ram and Trehan, 2010, p 421).

Information sharing by micros was also recognised and valued by the families of service users we spoke to, as illustrated by this family carer:

> *Carer:* That's why I'm very grateful for someone like [micro day service] to come along and for me to find out about this because it is proving to be very helpful.
> *Interviewer:* Mmm, and you were saying she knows about Social Services, she provides link to other things?
> *Carer:* Yes, ... she is very knowledgeable because I know she used to be a manager, I'm not quite sure in what area or where or anything like that, but yeah she's on the button with everything really by the seems of it." (Carer 222, Micro day service)

The next account, from two family carers of a person with physical and learning disabilities, displays why this type of informal information sharing offered by many micros is so valuable. The carers describe a difficult and lengthy process of identifying care services through a mainstream route.

> *Carer 1:* No, this is the frustrating part – they'll [leaflets] come from different day centres and 'well, we've never heard of it' [response from social worker], right, and if you work your way back it's down to the social worker to point you into the right direction, right. Well, I personally think some social workers have somebody favourite and some don't. Right, so unless you're pointed in –
> *Carer 2:* In the right direction – if you ask what's available, what's out there, well they just say 'well, there is nowhere' and that's what they told us isn't it? There is nowhere.
> *Carer 1:* We went to loads [of different services identified by the carers themselves] just trying it you know, and nothing, nothing seemed to suit until we hit on this one [a micro provider] and this one does." (Carers 209, Micro day service)

Our interviews with service users and carers suggested that 'word of mouth' and hearing at first hand about the positive experiences of others was the most common way for micro-enterprises to become visible to their end-users, especially where these accounts came from relatives. In the case of older people's services it was slightly more difficult to ascertain where information about micro-enterprises had come from, as many older people told us that one of their children had found out about the service they used. Our conversations with people using larger services did reflect a higher level of referrals from professionals such as nurses and social workers.

The importance of personal, word-of-mouth recommendations for achieving visibility of micro services suggests that small-scale personal networks are extremely important as a means to sustainability. This finding was also mentioned repeatedly when micro staff commented on the process of 'starting up' and bringing clients and families with them. This micro-enterprise manager voices her dependence on personal relationships and networks, along with the felt vulnerability of that situation:

> "Luckily I've generated new business because families know of me and have said [to the local authorities/social workers] 'excuse me, no, it's our first choice is [this micro day service] and if that doesn't work out then we would look

at the [local authority services]'. But that's only done not because I'm marketing but because of personal reputation and because of people who happen to know me and I can't really risk growing on such scanty threads." (Staff 106, Micro day service)

Several micro-enterprise staff complained that even if they did publicise through local authority channels, this didn't seem to bring new people to the service. For instance, one day service for BME women with disabilities explained how it had left leaflets in all the key council sites and it was included on the website as a suggested provider, but still even people who 'live round the corner' seemed to have no idea that it existed. A service for older people found a similar lack of response to being part of a formal network with its council and having website presence.

"Let me just say that, we don't get many referrals and that's something that we've looked at in a variety of different ways to push the service to work." (Staff 102, Micro one-to-one support)

The research team was given several examples of how local authorities gave out alphabetical lists of providers, leading some people simply to call the first one on the list, in the absence of any information about quality.

These observations indicate that in order to successfully integrate micro-enterprises into local care systems it may be necessary to move beyond inclusion on provider lists and towards a model of supported choice. Professionals (especially social workers) need to be actively aware of the options available and to talk about these options with service users and their families. There was a sense that at the moment this was not happening.

"So the social workers, what they'll do, they'll try all the big boys, then they'll go to the micros – so the big boys get the offers of work first." (Staff 103, Micro domiciliary care)

Peer-led organisations also have a strong role to play in relation to providing information and advice that supports choice (TLAP, 2009).

Financial viability

The distinctive financial context of micro-enterprises was discussed in Chapter Six. The data presented indicated that micro-enterprises did indeed offer better value for money: their hourly prices are on average lower than those of larger providers, while the outcomes achieved are better. However, there are other aspects of micro-enterprise financing that need to be taken into account when considering the viability of their financial model.

Our study revealed some concerns about the financial stability of some of the micro-enterprises. The pressure to keep rates competitive within the locality and the inability to service 'high value' packages with high staffing demands meant that some of the micro-enterprises were struggling to survive. People who initiate micro-enterprises often take a significant pay cut in real terms, especially those moving away from equivalent management roles in larger organisations. Starting up micro-enterprise care services was viewed as a gamble by many interviewees; something that required an entrepreneurial mindset as well as support, often provided by the local micro-enterprise coordinators. One person who had set up a micro-enterprise said:

> "Yeah, I don't think it would have been possible if I hadn't sort of completely ignored … the financial risk of what you're doing I suppose. Not in a careless way but certainly you've got to have a very sort of belief that at some point, you know, it's going to work." (Staff 303, Micro day service)

Micro-providers sometimes described absorbing the financial deficits as personal costs, especially in the initial phases of business development. One manager demonstrated clearly how their personal income fluctuations are used to provide flexibility for any financial shortcomings:

> "You don't want to think of it like a business but then you're thinking well if that money's not coming in how am I going to afford to pay the insurances and then, and it's just a constant worry, it really is. But we just end up taking less wages." (Staff 302, Micro day service)

According to another micro-enterprise:

"I've kept this going by my personal funds ... I've ploughed in money, so when we're not making money, I've propped it up. I think we're in our fourth year now. So I've put a lot of me into this and kept it going when, you know, we weren't making – you know, I haven't – there have been months – I've gone for six or seven months without drawing anything." (Staff 103, Micro domiciliary care)

Sustainability of care organisations is a factor that is increasingly being considered by national and local government as financial cuts to care services affect the viability of the whole sector (CQC/Institute of Public Care, 2014; Crawford and Read, 2015). There is evidence to show that a sudden change of care provider can be a distressing process for people who use the service, and one that counteracts the benefits that might be achieved during the life of the organisation (Scourfield, 2004). Our research was a snapshot of organisations at a single time point, rather than a longitudinal study that would have enabled us to see whether the organisations involved grew, folded or stayed the same size. But even over the few months of the fieldwork phase of the project, one of the micro-enterprises announced that it was closing down, citing insufficient clients and funds to continue trading.

The current focus on market failure as a response to declining public spending on care has spotlighted private residential providers, drawing attention to the impacts of the introduction of the National Living Wage (for example, Crawford and Read, 2015), with little exploration of the closure of smaller social care organisations. However, this study of micro-enterprises revealed that organisations with just a few members of staff also experience specific difficulties that can become serious threats to their sustainability. For organisations operating through just one or two key members of staff, absences have direct consequences on the services provided and need to be carefully planned. This partner in a micro-enterprise explains the difficulties of arranging cover to accommodate staff sickness and holiday leave:

"The buck stops with you at the end of the day. If there's something wrong then it's down to myself and my partner you know, so that's it. It seems like if you're sick you know, you've got to try and get in whether you're poorly or not. Touch wood we're lucky neither of us have been. Annual leave, taking a holiday can be difficult because you want people covering you that you trust." (Staff 203, Micro day service)

One of the larger micro-enterprises offered a specific service where it would cover for other micro-enterprises in the area if staff were sick or on holiday. As members of the local micro-enterprise forum they could let other micro-providers know about this service. ("And there's a lot of trust involved in this because the worst thing that could happen would be that we look after someone else's client, we do a fantastic job and then they want us to stay and then we are seen to have taken the client," said the manager of this organisation (Staff 103, Micro domiciliary care)). Some of the people using services had used this back-up provision and found it worked well.

Many micro providers we spoke to had not found solutions to staffing issues. For domiciliary services this often resulted in turning away certain types of client, people with the highest level of need, as there were insufficient staffing resources to provide the number of care hours needed. Several of the micro-enterprises gave examples of having to turn down work because they were unable to provide the 24-hour or multi-person support that was needed, further supporting this point. This fits with the account given by family carers in Chapter Eight about needing to look to larger providers when the frailty of their family member became more advanced. As one staff member said:

> "[T]he problem with buying care from a small business is that they haven't got the resources and they haven't got the back-up. That is the problem. And there is going to be the odd occasion where they'll say, 'I'm really sorry. I can't cover Sunday. You know, because we haven't got anyone'."
> (Staff 103, Micro domiciliary care)

This member of staff explains how clients are lost to larger providers in this way:

> "We were offered a client just before Christmas that we couldn't do, 'cause it was 24/7, two-to-one. I mean, we haven't got the staff to cover it … We don't do nights. We're not big enough … (Staff 103, Micro domiciliary care)

It was micro-organisations with two to five members of staff (that is, those that were not sole traders and had not crossed the threshold into being small) that appeared to find it most difficult to sustain themselves. The research found organisations that had grown beyond the micro in order to become sustainable, as well as those that were folding because they could not continue to operate on their existing resource base. This micro-provider of older people's day services describes their existence on the brink of sustainability:

> "'Well we don't make a profit. Basically it covers cost, yeah. I mean we've had to take a huge drop in wages but it kind of wasn't about that. As long as we could get a wage out of it you know, and it paid for itself, 'cos obviously you've got to pay for insurances and things like that." (Staff 302, Micro day activities)

Management of staff more generally was an issue for these micro-enterprises, as they sought to give staff sufficient hours to retain them, without leading to staff burn-out. Again, the sole traders had an advantage here, since their time imposed a limit on their activities (although some were working seven days a week, including some evenings).

Many of the micro-enterprises, whether sole traders or those with several staff, reported problems regarding lack of boundaries between home and work life. This included an unwillingness to say no to people, such that they were always on call.

> "Our mobiles are our business so even on holiday we cover phone calls and we don't turn anyone away just because we are on holiday. Sometimes people just need a natter." (Staff 109, Micro one-to-one support)

Staff also reported the difficulty of multi-tasking, of running a business while also being involved in the day-to-day provision of care. One founder of a micro-enterprise explained:

> "[T]here was a young gentleman I took on for about a year with severe learning disabilities ... And I'd be out with him ... for a coffee or whatever – 10-pin bowling – I'd be 10-pin bowling; my phone's ringing and it's either the council, potential clients, CQC, staff with problems, the accountant, and it's just not fair." (Staff 105, Micro one-to-one support)

Such problems were much less likely to be found in the small, medium and large providers, where managers are unlikely to be directly involved in front-line care provision.

Working with the local authority

The language of enterprise and care markets might be indicative of a context in which the state is less relevant to care provision, but this was not the case: the relationship between the micro-enterprises and the local authority continued to be a dominant factor in shaping the lived experiences of the micro-enterprises. Local authorities were the source of funding, hoped-for referrals and quality monitoring.

The financial and administrative complexity of dealing with the local authority was an ongoing frustration for many of the micro-enterprises.

> "So say, for example, that person is not entitled to the travel payment, we charge the city council but the city council charges the person, so it's all a bit disconnected because people will ring us and say 'oh you've sent us a bill for the transport', we say 'no, no, we don't send', unless it's a private pay person, you know, 'we've not sent you that, it's the city council'. Nobody knows what anybody's doing. It is very, very complicated." (Staff 305, Large day service)

Other financial barriers were generated by local authority processing of personal budgets. These included capped prices for services and the costing in of brokerage services, whether used or not. Processing payments from local authorities was also a barrier for micro-enterprises, with funds often taking a long time to reach the organisations. According to one micro-enterprise manager:

> "Well it's me that's doing it, you know, because you think well we're not big enough to have an administrator ... every time they say 'could you resend that invoice' ... I could paper the civic building with the copies of these invoices I've sent you, you know!" (Staff 205, Micro day service)

This was a particular issue for learning disabilities services, which were more likely than older people's services to be funded through personal budgets and direct payments. This micro-enterprise staff member talks about added complications for people who use services following changes to prices:

> "We put the price up, they have to go back to panel to have their budget increased or reallocated. So although it's their [personal] budget, the council is the administrator ...

> some of them manage their own money but, you know, a £3 increase means that they need to go back to get it approved.'" (Staff 205, Micro day service)

Most of the micro-enterprises were working with self-funders and direct payment holders, in part because local authority procurement rules effectively barred them from providing directly commissioned services. Although this exclusion was a barrier in terms of access to referrals – particularly for older people, who are more likely than people with learning disabilities to have their services directly commissioned – it did have advantages in terms of making the financial relationship more straightforward. Payment, for example, could be very swift.

> "We've got one guy who's brilliant, who's perhaps our biggest client. We see him two hours a day ... He lives near me and I walk his ... invoice down on the first of the month ... post it through early in the morning, and he'll pay me the same day ... through internet banking. We've got quite a battle going on, because one day ... I popped it through, popped into the shop to get a paper; he'd paid me by the time I got home." (Staff 103, Micro domiciliary care)

Even the large domiciliary provider in our study, which might be assumed to be the one benefitting from the administrative simplicity of high-volume local authority contracts, wanted to move more people onto direct payments so as to reduce its dependence on the local authority: "I would prefer them all to be direct payments and it's something that we're going to push for." It felt that this was a win–win for its organisation and the person providing support – by getting the local authority 'out of the way' it could provide more flexible care:

> "People can plan their lives and put their care in around them, you know, it's not so rigid. Generic home care sort of thing ... If they want a lie-in they can have a lie-in. If they want to go to bed later, they can. If they want to watch a film, things like that'." (Staff 113, Large domiciliary care)

This account very much fits with the overall rationale for the move to personalisation and personal budgets/direct payments. However, there are a couple of aspects of it which seemed more problematic. The first, although not directly articulated by any of the providers, is that late payments by self-funders and direct payment holders are easier for the companies to deal with: they can simply remove (or threaten to remove) the service until the bill is paid. Providers are less willing to place ultimatums on the local authority ("put my head above the parapet"). Particularly for large providers, the size of the contract with the local authority and the need to preserve relationships in anticipation of future rounds of tendering means that providers are reluctant to withdraw the service. From a business perspective, it is clearly problematic that local authority bills are not paid in a timely way, but for the people receiving care, it does insulate them from the direct financial risk of non-payment.

A second, related aspect is that the desire for more self-funders and direct payment holders was articulated by the large domiciliary care provider as being a way to get themselves more control in the process. Each time local authority contracts are put out to tender the local authority can take a certain percentage of clients off the current provider, but direct payment holders are excluded from this: "they are ours", in the words of the large provider. As well as this future financial benefit for the company, direct payment holders are also easier to work with because the company can set the terms of engagement.

> "Direct payments, we can say 'no, I'm sorry, we're not doing that', and then it's up to the client to find their own alternative … [whereas with local authority commissioned services] if somebody tried to cause trouble, if they played one staff against another, which does happen, you know we'd say to social services 'well we're not happy here because they are playing one staff against another' and [social services] say 'no, you've got to go in there'." (Staff 113, Large domiciliary care)

This opportunity to be more selective offers protection for the staff involved, but it may lead to the withdrawal of service for people perceived as being 'awkward' in some way. As before, the local authority involvement helps to ensure ongoing support, even for people who the agencies feel are difficult to care for.

As well as local authorities being a source of referrals, micro-enterprises look to them because they help to provide start-up advice and link micro-enterprises in with peers. The three localities in which we undertook the research were all areas in which the local authorities had been particularly active in supporting micro-enterprises to get started. In two of the localities, the micro-enterprises were part of local peer-support forums. This was an important part of building their identity as the local micro providers. It provided a space for learning about how others had overcome shared issues, such as registering with the CQC.

In some cases, however, the existence of a coordinator and a forum had established expectations that the local care context would be conducive to micro care provision, which was not necessarily the case, for the reasons set out above. For some micro-enterprises this created bitterness – "this area has a reputation for supporting micros, and it is an absolute load of rubbish" (Staff 103, Micro domiciliary care) – or at least frustration that large-scale care continued to be given so many advantages in the local care setting. One of the micro-enterprises said: "The council like big agencies, they can just make a phone call and put things in place." (Staff 106, Micro day service). At their most extreme, ineffective relationships with local authorities were seen to be slowing the development of both individual micro providers and the micro-enterprise sector. One micro-enterprise staff member described a conflict of interest for local authorities caught between utilising the 'market' of providers and promoting their own in-house provision:

> "It's been very difficult to move to any kind of pace really …
> because of [this locality's] policy currently of social workers
> only referring people to in-house services, because they've
> just set up their own in-house trading arm and families
> have been directed to that." (Staff 206, Micro day service)

Addressing some of the practical barriers that micro-enterprises encounter in working with local authorities seems to require further development of systems where individual service users can easily identify and commission their own services. This approach may be a viable alternative to localities attempting to set up commissioning contracts with a growing quantity of providers, many of which are too small to easily participate in tendering processes. A study of commissioning practices in relation to integrated care by Billings and de Weger (2015) found that a strong commitment and change of practice from local authorities is required to make micro providers visible to service users and accessible on equal terms with more well-known providers.

Quality and regulation

Few of the micro care providers had CQC registration. Such registration is required for organisations providing personal care (for example, help with washing and dressing). For most of the micro-enterprises either it was not required because of the low-level nature of the service or the cost and complexity of the process was prohibitive. Those that had gone for CQC registration felt that the process of getting registered had not been proportionate to their size of organisation: "We pay the same insurance and the same CQC licence as a much larger business" (Staff 103, Micro domiciliary care)

By not having CQC registration, micro-enterprises were limited in the range of activities they could undertake – and also were not able to use CQC reports as an indication of quality to potential clients. For some organisations, this lack of quality badging proved to be a specific barrier to attracting local authority and public confidence. Within the third sector in particular the establishment of kite-marks and membership in networks and associations are known to be powerful indicators of quality and distinction (Macmillan, 2012, p 14). In the three localities, there were discussions about how to assure the quality of micro-enterprises in the absence of CQC registration. In one area a quality mark – gold, silver or bronze – is awarded to micro-enterprises, based on compliance with procedures and feedback from people who have used the service. The quality rating appears in the local online directory so that people who use services, their carers or professionals are able to filter services based on their quality level. A local micro-enterprise coordinator explained how this gives people more information about the services:

'[I]t enables people on a direct payment [to] have more choice of choosing a quality service that's been assessed and monitored and they'll be monitored like we monitor our contracted service." (Micro-enterprise co-ordinator 102)

However, one of the people running a micro-enterprise described the process of attaining the badge as lengthy and intrusive:

"for us to go to the next level of the quality mark … it's unbelievable what they want us to do. Now, the other micros are all moaning about it but one or two of them will probably do it. And I've said no. After the year I've had, I'm not having them coming in, going through all our files. They want to see all the payroll records, they want to see my bank accounts, which are personal to me 'cause I'm a sole trader." (Staff 103, Micro domiciliary care)

Part of the narrative underlying the broader personalisation reforms was a critique of state-based measures of quality, and a call for more peer-based sharing of consumer information (In Control, no date b). This stems in part from the technology-inspired move to consumer rating systems in much of our service-sector interactions (with Trip Advisor being perhaps the best known). It also stems from a widespread sense that state-based quality standards – such as CQC ratings – have had limited impact on driving up quality within the sector (Public Accounts Committee, 2015). Micro-enterprises could benefit from the development of consumer-based measures of quality in localities. However, it is important to acknowledge that this type of information may not be accessible to or convincing for people who are not familiar with them from other aspects of their lives, suggesting that they can only ever be part of the answer to assuring the quality of care services.

Conclusion

Having looked at the visibility of micro-enterprises, their financial context, their interaction with the local authority and with the regulatory system, we can identify that enabling factors for micro-enterprises are connected to their ability to build partnerships and collaborations, particularly with the statutory sector, while maintaining their autonomy. Key barriers relate to access to potential users of the service, managing staff and making the financial aspects of running a business work in the cash-strapped, rule-bound context of care. These factors reinforce those found in other studies, but progress towards addressing them has been slow (DH and NAAPS, 2009).

Micro-enterprises often operate outside of local authority commissioning practices. In this study, micro-enterprises were selected in localities that are largely supportive of micro-enterprises and have some infrastructure in place to support them (including a micro-enterprise coordinator working with the local authority in each of the areas). Despite this, few micro-enterprises were receiving referrals from the local authority and some felt that commissioners continued to favour larger and more well-known care providers. Most found that word of mouth and local advertising was a more reliable route for gaining clients, which is known to be the way that many very small businesses establish a client base (Edwards and Ram, 2006, p 897). These routes may be adequate if people needing care have direct payments, and support to use them to make local care choices; however, the relatively low take-up of direct payments by older people highlights the need to provide alternative routes into micro-enterprise.

Some of the issues identified here relate to the advantages and disadvantages of running very small organisations, irrespective of whether they are care organisations or not. However, there are some themes that are distinctive to the care sector: the potential vulnerability of people who need support; the intimacy of the support given in the home; the labour-intensive nature of care work and its emotional intensity; the role of the local authority as the commissioner of care services; and the highly regulated nature of the sector. Some of these create particular opportunities for micro-enterprises, whereas others put a strain on people trying to operate at a micro scale.

ELEVEN

Conclusion: scaling down?

"How awful must it be to have strange faces creeping over your threshold on a regular basis?" (Staff 106, Micro day service)

This interview quote, from one of the micro-enterprise staff that we interviewed, is a fitting start to this concluding chapter, because it reaffirms the relational essence of care, the importance of being cared for and supported by someone familiar, and the anxieties of getting it wrong (Barnes et al, 2015). It also captures the distinctiveness of the home as a setting of particular significance: a place with a threshold separating it from the outside world in which the presence of strangers is particularly unsettling. The home is known to be a distinct site for care practices (Milligan, 2009) – although our interviews did also show the importance of secure and trusting relationships in community environments. The extent to which different care organisations are likely to be able to sustain such relationships was a key focus of our account of personalisation as enactment: what organisational conditions are likely to enable a person-centred service.

A crucial question that we have addressed in this book is whether micro-enterprises are better placed than larger organisations to meet this demand for person-centred care and support, based on secure and trusting relationships. Earlier chapters have outlined the findings from the research study in relation to the personalised care, improved outcomes and lower prices of micro-enterprises, and have considered what we learned from the local sites about which contextual factors help micro-enterprises to thrive. In this chapter we leave the focus on the research sites and look at the care system more broadly to consider the scope for micro-enterprises to become a more secure part of future social care provision.

The chapter suggests that care can be framed as a complex adaptive system, which has implications for the ways in which micro-enterprises can be supported and sustained. In particular it is recognised to be difficult for local authorities to shape and manage care markets because of the weakness of their coordinating tools. The chapter then goes on to suggest that, rather than seeing organisational growth as the best way to share the positive experiences of micro-enterprises, we should focus on non-replication forms of scaling, with networks of very small organisations sustaining each other. The next section takes the research findings about the importance of small scale and discusses how far it is possible for large organisations to embody the ethos and practices of smallness. The chapter also highlights ways forward for the research agenda, emphasising the value of comparative work across different geographies and longitudinal work to track the stability of such organisations over the long term.

Micro-enterprises within a care system

While the focus of much of the earlier chapters has been on measures of organisational effectiveness, it is also important to consider performance at a system level (Skelcher, 2008, p 28). Boyne highlights the importance of coordination across a system, when considering the literature on service improvement:

> Service improvement, in other words, may require more than higher effectiveness by individual organizations, or even by all organizations that are involved in providing a service. Improvement may not occur unless whole service delivery systems (including public, private and voluntary organizations) get better. (Boyne, 2003b, p 214)

The adult social care system in England, as in many other countries, involves a highly disparate set of institutions and actors, with weak coordination tools. One way to envision it is as a set of strata, each layered on the top of the other without removing the one underneath. Thus, state care was laid on top of familial care in the 20th century, while a large amount of care continued to be delivered by families. From the 1980s, private and third sector providers of care proliferated, taking away some of the state provision, but leaving some statutory services, particularly for people with more complex conditions. Micro-enterprises are arguably another layer on top of this, with the potential to provide some of the support currently being given by other providers, including families, but without wholly replacing any of the pre-existing layers.

The geological metaphor has an implicit temporal element: layers are added over time. Pollitt (2008) distinguishes between linear and cyclical metaphors of time, drawing on the work of Stephen Jay Gould (1988) to note the distinction between 'time as sequential, moving forwards like an arrow', and 'cycles or alternations' (Pollitt, 2008, pp 51–2). Whereas the build-up of strata suggests a linear progression of policy, it is also possible to argue that micro-enterprises are part of the cyclical turn of public policy, returning to quasi-familial and communal types of care that were replaced by industrial scales of care in the 19th and 20th centuries (Duffy, 2014). A hint of this is given in the romantic renderings of some accounts of small-scale care. Writing about Dutch health services, Postma draws attention to the utopian aspects of the small-scale, which in the media are contrasted with the 'monster of upscaling' (2015, p 100). A similar account could be given of the valorisation of the ways in which women are setting up micro-enterprises in their communities to offer care to people in ways akin to kinship: "You just do things for them as you would for your own parents, family" (Staff 101, Micro one-to-one support).

A third way of envisioning care is as a complex adaptive system (Bovaird, 2013, pp 168–9). Complexity theory is increasingly being used as an explanatory approach within public policy (Teisman and Klijn, 2008; Cairney, 2012). The distinctive contribution, as Cairney points out, is that 'we shift our analysis from individual parts of a system to the system as a whole; as a network of elements that interact and combine to produce systemic behaviour that cannot be broken down merely into the actions of its constituent parts' (Cairney, 2012, p 346). Such systems are characterised by a number of features, including a network of many agents acting in parallel, where control is highly dispersed and there are many shifting levels of organisations (Waldrop, 1994). Bovaird suggests that social care meets many of these conditions, given 'the way in which the market of social-care providers (both private and third sector) tends to be in constant flux' (Bovaird, 2013, p 169).

Most relevant to micro-enterprises in particular is the aspect of complex adaptive systems that there are 'many niches, each one of which can be exploited by an agent adapted to fill that niche' (Bovaird, 2013, p 164). As Bovaird argues, 'this is particularly evident in social care, where a wide variety of providers (often "spin outs" of staff and managers from "in-house" services) are constantly reshaping their organisational configuration and their services to win contracts from a wide variety of commissioners' (Bovaird, 2013, p 169). This point reprises the discussion in Chapter Two about the fluidity of organisational forms and the scope for modular organisations and clusters of innovative services to regroup in order to make their offer more appealing to resources holders.

In this kind of complex system, the challenge for government becomes one of coordination to ensure an adequate range and diversity of supply. This challenge is clearly at the forefront for many local government actors as they attempt to perform the market-shaping duties that are placed upon them by the Care Act 2014. As the Care Act guidance puts it, 'The ambition is for local authorities to influence and drive the pace of change for their whole market, leading to a sustainable and diverse range of care and support providers, continuously improving quality and choice, and delivering better, innovative and cost-effective outcomes that promote the wellbeing of people who need care and support' (DH, 2014, p 41). The language of the 'whole market' underscores that local authorities must not only oversee their directly provided services but should also play a more facilitative role in the broader care market, including services paid for through direct payments and purchased by self-funders.

Since the Care Act, a number of toolkits and guides have been produced to help local authorities take these steps, including *Commissioning for better outcomes: A route map* (LGA, 2015). However, many local authorities seem unsure about how to undertake these activities effectively. The complex interplay of factors outside of their control – from levels of demand to care regulation, workforce supply, wage structures and price limitations – makes it very difficult for local authorities to shape local markets. This is consistent with complexity theory, in which, as Cairney notes, 'The behaviour of complex systems is difficult (or impossible) to predict. They exhibit "non-linear" dynamics produced by feedback loops in which some forms of energy or action are dampened (negative feedback) while others are amplified (positive feedback). Small actions can have large effects and large actions can have small effects' (Cairney, 2012, p 347).

It may seem perverse to bring a whole-system perspective into a study that has focused on the meanings and behaviours of a particular set of actors within the care sector. However, as Cairney argues, this needs not be an either/or:

> there is scope to explore interpretive accounts of complexity
> if our aim is to understand how agents interpret, adapt to
> and influence their decision-making environment ... Such
> accounts would recognise the importance of agency and
> meaning, but also identify the limits to agency, when the
> actions of others – and factors beyond their control – limit
> their ability to act in particular ways. (Cairney, 2012, p 353)

This is what we have done in our research. In future work we plan to consider 'market shaping' from a systems perspective to explain how effectively local authorities are deploying their market-shaping duties. Bovaird (2008, p 324) highlights the likely limited impact of such activities, according to complexity theory:

> Planners and strategists will have lost their claim to 'superman' powers, which give them a pre-eminent role in guiding the local community towards the strategic high ground, the 'optimum' of economic and management fable. This approach deliberately eschews 'cause-and-effect' analysis, as it accepts that the agent is unlikely to be able to uncover the mainsprings of collective change within its own system. (Bovaird, 2008, p. 325)

Such fatalism is so at odds with the 'how to' tone of policy makers in relation to market shaping that it suggests a fruitful area for further study.

Scaling out?

This discussion links to the question of whether scaling up or scaling out is the most likely and effective strategy for micro-enterprises. Most of the micro-enterprises we spoke to did not envisage scaling up their operations, making them atypical of micro-businesses in other sectors (Ram and Trehan, 2010). The very small providers we spoke to feared losing their distinctive contribution and taking on the undesirable traits that they associated with larger care providers – care that was inflexible and depersonalised.

Nor were the micro-enterprises interested in becoming involved in consortia-type approaches, as sub-contractors working with large 'prime providers'. This model is increasingly common in parts of public services and is identified as a way to bring some of the insights and community connections of the 'social sector' into large-scale contracts (Crowe et al, 2015). However, the benefits in this for the small, third sector organisations are very uncertain. As Crowe et al note, 'Social sector organisations meanwhile rely increasingly on winning work from large private sector partners and some depend on these for their survival, creating lopsided partnerships' (Crowe et al, 2015, p 6). The most notorious example of this is the Work Programme, in which small sub-contracts have struggled to survive as the financial benefits of the consortium have been hoarded by prime contractors (Rees et al, 2012). Given that so many micro-enterprises have been set up by people with bad experiences of existing large care services – through working for those services or relying on them for care – it seems unlikely that they would greet opportunities for partnerships with such services with any enthusiasm. Certainly none of the organisations we interviewed discussed this as a strategy for the future.

To widen the benefits of micro-scale provision, without the perceived problems of scaling up and consortia arrangements, it may be that micro-enterprises could be involved in 'scaling out', also called 'non-replication scaling' (Bunt and Harris, 2010; Clark et al, 2012). This includes practices such as 'advocacy/policy models [and] movement-building models' (Clark et al, 2012, p 5). It suggests that micro-enterprises should offer peer support, speak at local events, write about their experiences, take part in research like ours and generally spread the word about what they have done and how others can do the same.

Clark et al note that much less is known about this kind of scaling than about the traditional forms of replication scaling:

> The literature on non-replication is clearly newer, less formalized, and less complete. Different writers are using different terminology to describe the same strategies, and their overlaps are not widely understood. There are very few case studies, almost no empirical studies, and thus very few tested or generalizable theories. It is an area still under consideration and lessons will continue to emerge. (Clark et al, 2012, p 6)

The data we gathered about micro-enterprises contributes to this emerging field.

This non-replication scaling is also about sharing the ideas and principles of micro-enterprise more broadly. As Major puts it, 'Growing impact doesn't necessarily require organizational growth or the wholesale replication of programs – it may instead require expanding an idea or innovation, technology or skill, advocacy or policy change' (Major, 2011, p 2). Research like our own micro-enterprise project plays a role here in ensuring that lessons about micro-enterprise can be learned and shared with policy makers at central and local government levels. There is further scope to develop the local networking aspects of micro-enterprises and to match up organisations for peer mentoring. Such activities do require a coordinating mechanism. The localities we worked in had a micro-enterprise coordinator to undertake this function – and, as Chapter Ten set out, the scope for micro activity to flourish in the absence of such a coordinator is limited. It also requires a willingness among micro-enterprises to be active members of a network and to be prepared to spend time spreading the word about what they do. The time limitations of this are apparent for people who are already working longer hours in their care work. However, one aspect that all the micro-enterprises we interviewed had in common was a desire to tell the story of their entrepreneurial journey: their disillusionment with existing care services, how they came to set up their organisation and how it had fared in its years of operation. In the staff interviews, we were able to say 'tell me about how you came to set up your agency', and in return heard lengthy, compelling and emotional accounts of their experience. This story-telling potential is one resource that micro-enterprises have already, and that could be harnessed and shared by local authorities looking to encourage more such organisations in their localities.

Scaling down?

Although a key finding from the research has been about the benefits associated with micro-enterprises, it is possible to distil this message down still further to the benefits of sustained relationships and holistic models of support. While in our research this approach was predominantly associated with micro-enterprises, here we consider the scope for larger organisations to learn from the micro model in their own care provision. It is unlikely that micro-enterprise alone will be able to satisfy the growing demand for social care, and there are likely to be some advantages to having a range of organisational types and sizes within the sector. Therefore the potential to share insights from the research with larger organisations is an important one.

The stimulus for this line of thinking came in part from the fieldwork, in which we were struck by what we learned from observing some of the larger organisations in our study. The first was a franchise of a large national chain. This organisation regularly wins national awards for the quality of its home care but is mainly used by self-funders, because its prices are high ('the Waitrose of social care', was how one local authority commissioner described it). The interviewee from this organisation was aware of the local micro-enterprise activity and explained that his organisation had tried to be part of it:

> "When we very first started we were invited along to the micro providers' meeting ... but of course once we explained who we were [a franchise] ... it was very apparent that we weren't a micro provider, which of course we're

not. But the sort of theories behind what lots of the micro providers do, I think are just as valid for large companies as they are for small." (Staff 112, Small domiciliary care)

This reflection prompted us to consider whether or not this claim could be sustained. Certainly the ethical approach to care articulated by this manager was very similar to that of the micro-enterprises, the staff retention rates were higher than the sector average and the people who used the service rated it highly. Some aspects of this are likely to be price based and, as pressures on costs intensify year on year, may never be attainable beyond affluent self-funders. This organisation provides calls for a minimum of one hour, for example, and staff are paid for travel time and fuel. But other aspects of its approach may have more transferable insights, for example in how staff are recruited.

"We set about ... by placing adverts in the sort of places where people who might have a skill as a care giver but hadn't been professional carers in the past might see them ... [T]he sort of people we're interested in are very often people who have been in a position where they've done care for their grandparents or their parents or relatives. Then sadly over the course of time that person's passed away, they've sat down after the event and thought, 'You know what? I was really good at that. I wonder if I can turn that into a job.' And in traditional care companies they can't or many of them can't because they haven't done care professionally before, and because lots of companies aren't prepared to invest in training people it means they want people who are already trained, ready to go and they can go out and provide the care yesterday." (Staff 112, Small domiciliary care)

The claim here, then, is that this company targets a different potential workforce than other care providers, and certainly the manager felt this was one reason why his service was rated so highly by the people using it. There is of course a cost aspect to this (investment in training), but it is also about more creative recruitment approaches that might not be more expensive. Lewis and West argue in favour of utilising older workers, critiquing the drive to push young people into care work without sensitivity to their suitability for it:

there is a tendency on the part of policymakers to think that carework can be done by anyone. Thus, the Centre for Workforce Intelligence (CWI, 2011) suggested that young and unemployed people should be encouraged to enter care work, despite evidence indicating that better quality care is associated with older, more experienced workers (Netten et al, 2007). (Lewis and West, 2014, p 12)

Of course experience has to be gained over time, but the approach set out above suggests that this need not be through formal care work, but can be through people's experience within their families.

The shift towards values-based recruitment as a complement to skills-based recruitment in a range of sectors is relevant here. Values-based recruitment is increasingly used in nursing, in particular in an attempt to address some of the apparent failings in compassion raised in the Francis Report into deaths at the Mid-Staffordshire Foundation Trust (Sawbridge and Needham, 2014). There is scope to explore whether it can be more widely used in a care setting, although an underlying premise of using such tools is that there is a labour market in which care organisations can be selective in whom they recruit, which may not be the case in some local economies when demand for labour outstrips supply. A high percentage of care workers in some areas of England are recent immigrants, which further complicates recruitment strategies (Lloyd, 2012). It is also a reminder of the complex ethics of care (Barnes et al, 2015), in which values can be discussed in relation to the person being supported, without necessarily being sensitive to values in relation to care workers: 'Older people in high income countries might be able to exercise choice to have personalised services in their own homes, but their choice is made possible by the migration of low-paid workers from low and middle income countries to carry out the work' (Lloyd, 2012, p 126).

A second large organisation that we encountered during the research that is worthy of further consideration is a national charity providing accommodation for people with learning disabilities. Like many large organisations in the care sector it operates from a series of self-managing local bases. The approach to service delivery is particularly concerned with scale – creating small personal support networks around individuals. People who were housed by the service invoked the same sense of closeness and trust as the micro care service users. The importance of the service to this interviewee's life is clear:

"I actually shudder to think what would – what I'd be like if
I didn't have [care service, national charity]. They've helped
me improve and change so much, and they've helped me
actually create, you know, a proper life. Like, I have my own
house, now, and basically I've got all my own freedom. I can
have – basically, if I've got any concerns, they're just there
to help me with whatever I need. And they've improved
my life drastically and, you know, I know for a fact they're
doing it for many other people, as well." (Person with
learning disabilities 231, Large accommodation service)

What seems to be distinctive here is the commitment to creating
a reliable and friendly environment for people with social care
needs. After people have been housed the charity continues to
support residents by building networks of volunteers and links to the
community and offering as much personal support as its users feel they
need. An implicit aim for this charity that is not always as evident in
the work of other micro-enterprises is the goal of making clients less
dependent on it over time. Of course this may be more achievable for
younger users' groups than it is for frail older people.

A third model to consider is how far a large service can be a hub
for micro-enterprise activity, which was how one of the large local
authority day centres in our study saw its future. Across the UK, local
authorities are being encouraged to develop 'community hubs' that
can be the locus for 'personalised activities and learning opportunities'
(Carr, 2010, p vii). Such places are often counterpoised to existing day
centres – framed as outdated, segregated and unfit for purpose – with
hubs instead 'promis[ing] a "win win" future of new shared spaces'
(Needham, 2014, p 104). There has been suspicion that this agenda
is simply a way to draw attention away from widespread day centre
closures that are driven more by financial pressures than by the likely
emergence of a network of thriving community hubs (Roulstone and
Morgan, 2009; Mencap, 2012; Needham, 2014). A potential insight
from our research is that day centres (where not already closed down)
could make use of their building space to provide facilities from which
micro-enterprises could operate. This, then, is a nested model, in which
micros 'piggy back' on a larger provider, renting space and accessing
a larger population of potential service users than is possible when
operating out of a home office.

Outside of this study we have come across other large organisations
that are trying to harness some of the insights of small-scale working,
particularly with regard to staff autonomy and creativity. A prominent

example of an organisation that seems to be able to harness the benefits of a small-scale relational approach on a large scale is Buurtzorg in the Netherlands (Laloux, 2014; Gray et al, 2015). This home care provider has 8,000 nurses providing care across the country. However, they all work in self-managed teams of 10–12 people, with no management outside the team (although coaches are available). Each team supports around 50 patients within a neighbourhood. The Buurtzorg model emphasises a holistic type of care in which highly trained nurses help with everything that is needed by a frail older person or a person with a long-term health condition or disability. Thus, nurses will dress bandages and dispense medicines, but they will also hang out washing and link people up with their neighbours. As Laloux (2014, pp 65–6) writes:

> Care is no longer fragmented. Whenever possible, things are planned so that a patient always sees the same one or two nurses. Nurses take time to sit down, drink a cup of coffee, and get to know the patients and their history and preferences ... Care is no longer reduced to a shot or a bandage – patients can be seen and honoured in their wholeness, with attention paid not only to their physical needs, but also their emotional, relational, and spiritual ones ... Nurses will often go ring at a neighbor's door to inquire if they would be open to helping support the older lady living next door. Buurtzorg effectively tries to make itself redundant whenever possible.

Evaluation of Buurtzorg has shown it to be effective in relation to outcomes and value for money, and other countries are now experimenting with the Buurtzorg model (Gray et al, 2015). Its integration of health and social care could be a good fit in a UK setting in which such integration remains a much sought-after policy goal (DH, 2014). We use it here as further support for the argument that the benefits of smallness need not necessarily be lost when organisations scale up, so long as small, autonomous units are preserved.

The politics of micro-enterprise

This book has been about whether, how and why micro-enterprises can provide individuals and families with high-quality, personalised, innovative and affordable social care. Our conclusion – that micro-enterprises can make a high-quality contribution to care provision that offers better value for money and more person-centred support – has implications for how care is commissioned. Our data suggests that a growth in micro care provision requires more people to have a personal budget in order to commission micro support themselves, given the difficulties that local authorities have in working well with a multiplicity of very small organisations. This finding has a political dimension that needs to be acknowledged. The introduction suggested that micro-enterprise could be considered a form of new left, community-based provision, and that political opposition to the micro-enterprises could be characterised as expressive of 'old left' advocacy of state-based solutions. It is of course also possible to give other readings, of which the most prevalent is that micro-enterprises and personal budgets together constitute the apogee of a neoliberal model of privatised social care. In this account it is the financialised individual who takes responsibility for buying care and bears the risks of things going wrong (Burchell, 1996). It is a step closer to the personal voucher state that elements of the Conservative Party have long advocated (Joseph, 1975; Carswell and Hannan, 2008).

It is certainly the case that a proliferation of very small providers will make it difficult for government to monitor and assure the quality that is provided. It may contribute to the development of a fragmented market that can best be navigated by those who are well informed, resourced and networked. Accountability of providers to service users may also be an issue if lots of small, and potentially fluid and unstable, organisations replace a small number of larger providers. However, it is important to be aware that the existing large organisations are also unaccountable and unstable, with much higher failure risks for local care systems than are implied by the disappearance of a micro-enterprise (Campbell, 2015).

There clearly remains a role for the state in overseeing care markets and providing access to information and support that can mitigate equity concerns. Writing more broadly about innovation, the economist Mazzucato (2013) affirms that the state will continue to have a role in supporting innovation, as it has done in the past. Similarly we envisage a context in which the state remains an active partner in shaping adult social care. Micro-enterprises are a large part of existing care markets (up to a third of care providers, based on Skills for Care data (2015)). However, growth in the sector is coming from very large providers (CQC, 2015), suggesting that not enough is being done to support micro-level care. As well as the broader vulnerabilities of micro businesses (with their very high failure rate), micro care providers are particularly reliant on local authorities in the ways discussed in Chapter

Ten. Understanding how to provide support as part of a broader commitment to market shaping under the Care Act is a real challenge for local authorities.

However, the political challenge here goes beyond simply adding micro-enterprises to the menu of social care services. The dramatic scale of the cuts to care services creates an existential threat to many current providers, and leaves many older and disabled people at risk of inadequate support. Personalisation, which came with promises of cost savings, can in no way ameliorate cuts of this scale and risks being left exposed as the justification for cuts that lack any other kind of legitimising narrative (West, 2013; Needham, 2014). This setting puts enormous and unsustainable pressures on people working within care services. Steckley (2015, p 199) observes that many social workers and managers work in a social and political context 'which mitigate[s] their alertness, or attentiveness, to barely acceptable situations for older people'. Steckley goes on to invoke Bauman's (2006) concept of adiaphorisation that 'leads to an ethical deskilling of workers by desensitising their moral sensibilities and repressing their moral urges' (Steckley, 2015, p 199).

As well as the toll this takes on staff, managers and the people receiving care and their families, the broader political context must remain in view. Barnes et al (2015, p 235) call for a political response that is rooted in a feminist ethic of care:

> Neither developing individual virtues of compassion, nor arguing for collective responsibility without recognising the impact of structural disadvantage and the profoundly oppressive nature of unequal social relations, can deliver the transformative objectives of feminist care ethics. Without an explicitly political stance, arguments for prioritising care can be safely taken on board within the existing power structures and comfortably accommodated in regressive political agendas.

These authors suggest that 'an explicit adoption of a care ethics language and perspective could provide a starting point for a dialogue about what constitutes good care' (Barnes et al, 2015, p 241). Again it seems to us that micro-enterprises can make a contribution here, with an ethic of care sitting well with the articulation of enacted personalisation – but only as part of a broader political debate about how we design and fund care that enhances dignity and personhood.

Skelcher asks: 'So what is the "best" form of governance? This is a question that can only be answered by understanding the predominant discourse applying in a particular context' (Skelcher, 2008, p 41). The care sector is dominated by twin discourses: one of person-centred care; the other of cuts and crisis. The organisations that to us seem most likely to be able to deliver on the first discourse and survive the second are the micro-enterprises we encountered, provided that both national and local government work to support their contribution. The market-shaping capacities of local authorities, set down in the Care Act 2014, are still very underdeveloped. Large local authorities like to contract with large care agencies because the common scale creates an organisational match. Procurement processes and referral patterns are ill-suited to small-scale provision. Yet, if the future of care services is not simply to be a series of crisis-driven responses to the failure of large residential and domiciliary care providers, local authorities need to act now to encourage community-based, small-scale provision.

Where next for micro-enterprises and the research agenda?

Micro-enterprises in social care are already making a significant contribution to care and support, and the research developed here suggests that this should continue. More needs to be known about how local authorities can develop local care markets as settings in which a diverse range and size of providers can thrive. Further research could illuminate the different patterns of provision and success in micro-enterprises in different geographic jurisdictions. Scotland and Wales are both pursuing forms of self-directed care that differ from the approach taken in England – there is more in-house provision of care, for example, and less appetite for market-type solutions (Gray and Birrell, 2013). Micro-enterprises could thrive in this setting in so far as they are associated with dominant themes regarding community co-production of services; but not if they are seen as market alternatives to state provision (Pearson et al, 2014). Comparative research beyond the UK again can usefully highlight the different types of narrative with regard to scale – as Postma's (2015) work has done in the Dutch case – and the ways in which these are manifest in care systems.

Future research on micro-enterprises would most usefully take a longitudinal perspective. Our research was a snapshot of service provision at a particular time. As such, we were unable to capture the changing nature of local care markets and the extent to which micro-enterprises were stable providers within it. We know from many of our interviews that the micro-providers were financially precarious, and indeed one of our case study organisations ceased trading before our research was complete. But we know also that question marks hang over a lot of large providers at the time when we are writing, and that the collapse of a large-scale organisation wreaks much more devastation than that of a very small organisation. Understanding the dynamics of care providers over a long term would help to give a better sense of what features are associated with survival within a care system, and how local authorities can better reinforce these survival factors (Macmillan, 2011; Macmillan et al, 2013).

Conclusion

The book has used micro-enterprises to consider a range of research themes that have widespread implications: the relationship between organisational size and performance in a care setting, and how this intersects with the costs of care; the enactment of personalised care, and the extent to which there are organisational characteristics that support this enactment; the different types of innovation that are at work in a care setting, and the ways in which innovation maps onto organisational size. These contributions are primarily to academic debates within social policy and public management. As we acknowledged earlier in the book, our contributions are to theorising the relationships between size, performance and innovation in a care setting, not to making statistical generalisations. In relation to micro-enterprises, then, this suggests that our work contributes to stronger theorisation of the benefits of small-scale approaches to care that future work can build on.

We have also offered policy-relevant findings about the advantages that micro-enterprises bring to local care settings, and the factors that can limit their impact. The care sector is in a more precarious state as we finish this book than it was when we started the research, and the palpable sense of despair within the sector makes it a difficult setting in which to make any kinds of utopian claims. We don't suggest that micro-enterprises can solve the underfunding of social care, but we do argue that they offer the best hope for sustaining person-centred services on a tight budget. The economies of scale offered by large-scale care providers may look alluring, but recent history would suggest that such siren calls are best resisted: they undercost the service, imposing working conditions on staff that are antithetical to person-centred care. The solution to this is not merely more clever contracting – turning to outcomes-based commissioning approaches, for example, as the salvation of large-scale contracting. As we quoted Bovaird in Chapter

Six, outcomes are often chosen because they are 'easy to measure, fashionable, or sympathetically regarded by the controlling political group' (Bovaird, 2012, pp 4–5). Good care is relational, it is a process not an outcome, and our research supports others who have found that it is most likely to happen where staff have autonomy, flexibility and the scope to build up sustained relationships with the people they care for (Lewis and West, 2014; Eldh et al, 2015). All of these things are more likely to occur when care is on a small scale.

Appendix 1: Site one interview schedule

Micro-enterprise project
Interview questions

Part 1: Getting started

1. Introductions – tell people your name and circumstances/experiences. Explain why there are two interviewers
2. Ask interviewee to introduce themselves. [*Maybe ask about family photos to break the ice*]
3. Explain the project briefly and ask them to fill in and sign the **consent form**
4. Ask if they have got any questions before we start

Part 2: Interview

We are primarily interested in the care and support you get from [Care service].

1. How long have you been receiving services from [Care service]?
2. What support did you have previously (if any)? How does [Care service] compare to this?
3. What services does [Care service] provide for you?
4. Do you get much choice about what support you get AND who provides it?
5. Is it usually the same person who provides it? Do you call that person by their first name?
6. Do you use other paid service providers or just [Care service]?
7. Did you choose [Care service] or did someone else choose it? Why did you/they choose [Care service]? How did you/they hear about [Care service]?
8. What, if anything, do you like about what [Care service] provides? Can you give us an example of something that has worked well?
9. What, if anything, don't you like about what they provide? Can you give us an example of something that hasn't worked well?

10. What would be a good day for you? How often do you have that kind of a day? Does [Care service] play a role in helping that happen?
11. Would you recommend [Care service] to family and friends who needed similar support?
12. Do you mind me asking, do you pay for [Care service] yourself or does the council pay?
13. Do you think [Care service] are good value for money?
14. Is there anything else you would like to tell us about [Care service]?

Part 3: ASCOT survey

We have a few survey questions to ask you before we finish if that's OK ...

Part 4: End of interview

1. Thanks for your time.
2. We will send you a copy of our final report and let you know if we are organising any events locally that you might like to come along to.
3. Do you have any final questions?

Appendix 2: Adapted ASCOT tool

Q1: Occupation

1a. Do you do things you value and enjoy with your time?

Please tick (☑) one box

I'm able to spend my time as I want, doing things ☐
I value or enjoy (4)

I'm able to do enough of the things I value or ☐
enjoy with my time (3)

I do some of the things I value or enjoy with my ☐
time but not enough (2)

I don't do anything I value or enjoy with my ☐
time (1)

1b. Do the support and services that you get from <<EXAMPLE>>
affect how you spend your time?

Please tick (☑) one box

Yes (1) ☐

No (0) ☐

Don't know (2) ☐

1c. Imagine that you didn't have the support and services from
<<EXAMPLE>> that you do now and no other help stepped in. In
that situation, which of the following would best describe how you
spend your time?

Please tick (☑) one box

I would be able to spend my time as I want, ☐
doing things I value or enjoy (4)

I would be able do enough of the things I value or enjoy with my time (3) ☐

I would do some of the things I value or enjoy with my time but not enough (2) ☐

I wouldn't do anything I value or enjoy with my time (1) ☐

Q2: Control over daily life

2a. Do you feel you have control over your daily life?

> **Interviewer prompt**: *By 'control over daily life' we mean having the choice to do things or have things done for you as you like and when you want*

Please tick (☑) one box

I have as much control over my daily life as I want (4) ☐

I have adequate control over my daily life (3) ☐

I have some control over my daily life but not enough (2) ☐

I have no control over my daily life (1) ☐

2b. Do the support and services that you get from <<EXAMPLE>> affect how much control you have over your daily life?

Please tick (☑) one box

Yes (1) ☐

No (0) ☐

Don't know (2) ☐

2c. Imagine that you didn't have the support and services from
<<EXAMPLE>> that you do now and no other help stepped in.
In that situation, which of the following would best describe the
amount of control you'd have over your daily life?

Please tick (☑) one box

I would have as much control over my daily life ☐
as I want (4)

I would have adequate control over my daily ☐
life (3)

I would have some control over my daily life ☐
but not enough (2)

I would have no control over my daily life (1) ☐

Interviewee ID: _____
☐ **Older Person (1)**   ☐ **Learning Disability (2)**

Age:
☐ 18-25 (1)   ☐ 26-35 (2)   ☐ 36-45 (3)   ☐ 46-55 (4)
☐ 56-65 (5)   ☐ 66-75 (6)   ☐ 76-85 (7)   ☐ Over 85 (8)

Gender: ☐   Male (1)   ☐   Female (2)

Marital Status:
☐ Married (1)   ☐ Co-habiting (2)   ☐ Widowed (3)
☐ Divorced (4)   ☐ Single (5)
☐ Other (6) _____

Ethnic Group:
☐ White (British, Irish, or any Other White background) (1)
☐ Black or Black British (Caribbean, African or any Other Black background) (2)
☐ Mixed (White/Black Caribbean, White/Black African, White/Asian, or other mixed background) (3)
☐ Chinese (4)
☐ Asian or Asian British (Indian, Pakistani, Bangladeshi, or any other Asian background) (5)
☐ Any other ethnic group (6) _____

Area of Residence:
- ☐ Site 1 urban (1)
- ☐ Site 1 rural (2)
- ☐ Site 2 urban (3)
- ☐ Site 2 rural (4)
- ☐ Site 3 urban (5)
- ☐ Site 3 rural (6)

Name of care provider: _____

Appendix 3: Developing the innovation theme codes

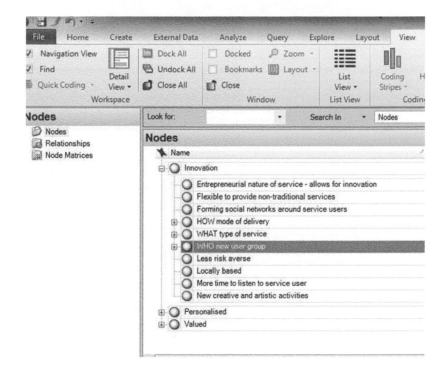

References

ACEVO (Association of Chief Executives of Voluntary Organisations) (2010) *How to cost appropriately with personal budgets*, London: ACEVO.

Ackroyd, S. and Karlsson, J.C. (2014) 'Critical realism as an empirical project', in P.K. Edwards, J. O'Mahoney and S. Vincent (eds) *Studying organizations using critical realism*, Oxford: Oxford University Press, pp 21–45.

Age UK (2013) *Making managed personal budgets work for older people*, London: Age UK, www.ageuk.org.uk/professional-resources-home/services-and-practice/care-andsupport/personalisation-hub/making-personal-budgets-work-for-older-people/ (accessed 17 January 2014).

Aiken, M., Bacharach, S.B. and French, J.L. (1980) 'Organizational structure, work process, and proposal making in administrative bureaucracies', *Academy of Management Journal*, vol 23, pp 631–52.

Alcock, P. (2010) 'Building the Big Society: a new policy environment for the third sector in England', *Voluntary Sector Review*, vol 1, no 3, pp 379–89.

Andrews, R., Boyne, D.G., Law, J. and Walker, R.M. (2012) *Strategic management and public service performance*, Basingstoke: Palgrave Macmillan.

Archer, R. (1989) 'Introduction', in R. Archer (ed) *Out of apathy, voices of the New Left 30 years on*, London: Verso, pp 1–10.

Attride-Stirling, J. (2001) 'Thematic networks: an analytic tool for qualitative research', *Qualitative Research*, vol 1, no 3, pp 385–405.

Barnes, M. (2012) *Care in everyday life: An ethic of care in practice*, Bristol: The Policy Press.

Barnes, M., Brannelly, T., Ward, L. and Ward, N. (2015) *Ethics of care: Critical advances in international perspective*, Bristol: The Policy Press.

Bauman, Z. (2006) *Liquid fear*, Cambridge: Polity Press.

Baxter, K., Glendinning, C. and Greener, I. (2011) 'The implications of personal budgets for the home care market', *Public Money and Management*, March, pp 91–9.

Behn, R.D. (2003) 'Why measure performance? Different purposes require different measures', *Public Administration Review*, vol 63, no 5, pp 86–606.

Bennett, R. and Gabriel, H. (2003) 'Image and reputational characteristics of UK charitable organizations: an empirical study', *Corporate Reputation Review*, vol 6, pp 276–89.

Beresford, P. (2007) 'The role of service user research in generating knowledge-based health and social care: from conflict to contribution', *Evidence and Policy*, vol 3, no 4, pp 329–41.

Beresford, P. (2008) 'Whose personalisation?' *Soundings*, vol 40, Winter, pp 8–17.

Bhaskar, R.A. (1997) [1975] *A realist theory of science*, London: Verso.

Bhaskar, R.A. (1998) [1979] *The possibility of naturalism* (3rd edn), London: Routledge.

Bickerstaffe, S. (2013) *Towards whole person care*, London: IPPR, www.ippr.org/publication/55/11518/towards-whole-person-care (accessed 4 February 2014).

Billings, J. and de Weger, E. (2015) 'Contracting for integrated health and social care: a critical review of four models', *Journal of Integrated Care*, vol 23, no 3, pp 53–175.

Birch, R.C. (1974) *The shaping of the welfare state*, Harlow: Longman.

BIS (Department for Business, Innovation and Skills) (2010) *Business, start ups and economic churn: A literature review*, London: NIESR.

Blaikie, N. (2009) *Designing social research* (2nd edn), Cambridge: Polity Press.

Bolton, S.C. and Wibberley, G. (2013) 'Domiciliary care: the formal and informal labour process', *Sociology*, vol 48, no 4, pp 682–97.

Bovaird, T. (2008) 'Emergent strategic management and planning mechanisms in complex adaptive systems', *Public Management Review*, vol 10, no 3, pp 319–40.

Bovaird, T. (2012) 'Attributing outcomes to social policy interventions – "gold standard" or "fool's gold" in public policy and management?' *Social Policy and Administration*, vol 48, no 1, pp 1–23.

Bovaird, T. (2013) 'Context in public policy: implications of complexity theory', in C. Pollitt (ed) *Context in public policy and management: The missing link?* Cheltenham: Edward Elgar, pp 157–77.

Bowes, A.M. and Dar, N.S. (2000) 'Researching social care for minority ethnic older people: Implications of some Scottish research', *British Journal of Social Work*, vol 30, no 3, pp 305–21.

Boyle, D. (2011) *The human element*, London: Routledge.

Boyle, D. and Murphy, M. (2009) *A better return: Setting the foundations for intelligent commissioning to achieve value for money*, London: New Economics Foundation.

Boyne, G.A. (1996) 'Scale, performance and the new public management: an empirical analysis of local authority services', *Journal of Management Studies*, vol 33, pp 809–26.

Boyne, G.A. (2002) 'Theme: Local government: concepts and indicators of local authority performance: an evaluation of the statutory frameworks in England and Wales', *Public Money and Management*, vol 22, no 2, pp 17–24.

Boyne, G.A. (2003a) 'Sources of public service improvement: a critical review and research agenda', *Journal of Public Administration Research and Theory*, vol 13, pp 367–94.

Boyne, G.A. (2003b) 'What is public service improvement?' *Public Administration*, vol 81, no 2, pp 211–27.

Brandsen, T. and Pestoff, V. (2006) 'Co-production, the third sector and the delivery of public services', *Public Management Review*, vol 8, no 4, pp 493–501.

Brindle, D. (2008) *Care and support: A community responsibility?* York: Joseph Rowntree Foundation.

British Psychological Society (2009) *Code of Ethics and Conduct: Guidance published by the Ethics Committee of the British Psychological Society*, Leicester: The British Psychological Society

Brown, K. (2015) *Vulnerability and young people: Care and social control in policy and practice*, Bristol: The Policy Press.

Bruner, J. (1986) *Actual minds, possible worlds*, Cambridge, MA: Harvard University Press.

Bubb, S. and Michell, R. (2009) 'Investing in third sector capacity', in P. Hunter (ed) *Social enterprise for public service: How does the third sector deliver?* London: The Smith Institute, pp 74–83.

Buckingham, H. (2012) 'Capturing diversity: a typology of third sector organisations' responses to contracting based on empirical evidence from homelessness services', *Journal of Social Policy*, vol 41, no 3, pp 569–89.

Bunt, L. and Harris, M. (2010) *Mass localism: A way to help small communities solve big social challenges*, London: NESTA.

Burchell, G. (1996) 'Liberal government and techniques of the self', in A. Barry, T. Osborne and N. Rose (eds) *Foucault and political reason: Liberalism, neo-liberalism and rationalities of government*, London: UCL Press, pp 19–36.

Burstow, P. (2014) *Key to care: Report of the Burstow Commission on the future of the home care workforce*, London: Local Government Information Unit, www.lgiu.org.uk/2014/12/02/key-to-care-report-of-the-burstow-commission-on-the-future-of-the-home-care-workforce/ (accessed 7 April 2016).

Butler, J. (1993) *Bodies that matter: On the discursive limits of 'sex'*, London: Routledge.

Cabinet Office (1999) *Modernising government*, London: HMSO.

Cabinet Office (2010a) 'Government launches Big Society programme', https://www.gov.uk/government/news/government-launches-big-society-programme--2 (accessed 12 October 2015).

Cabinet Office (2010b) *Building the Big Society*, London: Cabinet Office, www.cabinetoffice.gov.uk/media/407789/building-big-society.pdf (accessed 12 October 2015).

Caiels, J., Forder, J., Malley, J., Netten, A. and Windle, K. (2010) *Measuring the outcomes of low-level services: Final report*, University of Kent: Personal Social Services Research Unit, www.pssru.ac.uk/pdf/dp2699.pdf (accessed 25 January 2012).

Cairney, P. (2012) 'Complexity theory in political science and public policy', *Political Studies Review*, vol 10, pp 346–58.

Callon, M. (2007) 'What does it mean to say that economics is performative?', in D. MacKenzie, F. Muniesa and L. Siu (eds) *Do economists make markets? On the performativity of economics*, Princeton: Princeton University Press.

Cambridge, P., Hayes, L., and Knapp, M. with Gould, E. and Fenyo, A. (1994) *Care in the community: Five years on*, Canterbury: Personal Social Services Research Unit, University of Kent.

Camison Zornoza, C., Lapiedra-Alcamí, C., Segarra-Ciprés, M. and Boronat-Navarro, M. (2004) 'A meta-analysis of innovation and organizational size', *Organization Studies*, vol 25, no 3, pp 331–61.

Campbell, D. (2015) 'Half of UK care homes will close unless £2.9bn funding gap is plugged, charities warn', *Guardian*, 21 November, www.theguardian.com/society/2015/nov/21/half-uk-care-homes-close-funding-gap-nhs-george-osborne (accessed 21 November 2015).

Carr, S. (2010) *Personalisation, productivity and efficiency*, Research briefing 37, London: Social Care Institute for Excellence.

Carr, S. and Robbins, D. (2009) *SCIE Research Briefing 20: The implementation of individual budget schemes in adult social care*, London: SCIE.

Carswell, D. and Hannan, D. (2008) *The plan: Twelve months to renew Britain*, London: Carswell.

CWI (Centre for Workforce Intelligence) (2011) *Workforce risks and opportunities: Adult social care*, London: CWI.

Chapain, C., Cooke, P., De Propris, L., MacNeill, L. and Mateos-Garcia, J. (2010) *Creative clusters and innovation: Putting creativity on the map*, London: National Endowment for Science, Technology and the Arts.

Clark, C., Massarsky, C., Raben, T. and Worsham, E. (2012) *Scaling social impact: A literature toolkit for funders*, Durham, NC: Duke University/Growth Philanthropy Network.

Clarke, J., Cochrane, A. and Smart, C. (1987) *Ideologies of welfare: From dreams to disillusion*, London: Hutchinson.

Community Catalysts (no date) *Micro enterprise: Harnessing community capacity to deliver great outcomes and savings*, Wythall: In Control, www.in-control.org.uk/media/106733/micro%20enterprise.pdf.

Community Catalysts (2011) *Enterprise for all: Care or community support services run by people who have experienced them: a practical guide for enterprising people*, Harrogate: Community Catalysts.

Community Catalysts (2014) *Microenterprise*, www.communitycatalysts.co.uk/products/micro-enterprise/ (accessed 12 February 2015).

Commission for Social Care Inspection (2006) *The state of social care in England 2005–06*, London: Commission for Social Care Inspection.

Commission on Funding of Care and Support (2011) *Fairer care funding – The report of the Commission on Funding of Care and Support*, London: The Stationery Office.

Considine, M. (2000) 'Selling the unemployed: the performance of bureaucracies, firms and non-profits in the new Australian "market" for unemployment assistance', *Social Policy and Administration*, vol 34, no 3, pp 274–95.

Corbin, J and Strauss, A (1990) 'Grounded theory research: Procedures, canons, and evaluative criteria', *Qualitative Sociology*, vol 13, Issue 1, pp 3–21

Cottam, H. (2009) 'Public service reform, the individual and the state', *Soundings*, vol 42, pp 79–89.

CQC (Care Quality Commission) (2015) *The state of health care and adult social care in England 2014/15*, London: Care Quality Commission, www.cqc.org.uk/sites/default/files/20151103_state_of_care_web_accessible_4.pdf (accessed 21 November 2015).

CQC/Institute of Public Care (2014) *The Stability of the care market and market oversight in England*, Oxford: Oxford Brookes University, www.cqc.org.uk/sites/default/files/201402-market-stability-report.pdf (accessed 7 April 2016).

Crawford, E. and Read, C. (2015) *The care collapse: The imminent crisis in residential care and its impact on the NHS*, Interim Report, ResPublica, www.respublica.org.uk/wp-content/uploads/2015/11/ResPublica-The-Care-Collapse (accessed 11 November 2015).

Crowe, D., Gash, T. and Kippin, H. (2015) *Beyond big contracts: Commissioning public services for better outcomes*, London: Collaborate at South Bank University.

Cunningham, I. and James, P. (2007) *False economy? The costs of contracting and workforce insecurity in the voluntary sector*, London: Unison.

Curran, J. (1990). 'Rethinking economic structure: exploring the role of the small firm and self-employment in the British economy', *Work, Employment and Society*, vol 4, pp 125–46.

Currie, G., Ford, J., Harding, N. and Learmonth, M. (eds) (2010) *Making public services management critical*, London: Routledge.

Czarniawska, B. (1997) 'A four times told tale: combining narrative and scientific knowledge in organization studies', *Organization*, vol 4, no 1, pp 7–30.

Daft, R. and Becker, S.W. (1978) *Innovation in organizations*, New York: Elsevier.

Dahler-Larsen, P. (2005) 'Evaluation and public management', in E. Ferlie, L. Lynn and C. Pollitt (eds) *The Oxford Handbook of Public Management*, Oxford: Oxford University Press, pp 615–42.

Daly, M. (2013) 'Juicing, dancing and sewing: how micro-providers are adding colour to personalisation', *Community Care*, www.communitycare.co.uk/2013/06/10/juicing-dancing-and-sewing-how-micro-providers-are-adding-colour-to-personalisation/#.UvykHPl_t0o (accessed February 2014).

Damanpour, F. (1992) 'Organizational size and innovation', *Organization Studies*, vol 13, pp 375–402.

Damanpour, F. (1996) 'Organizational complexity and innovation: developing and testing multiple contingency models', *Management Science*, vol 42, no 5, pp 693–713.

Damanpour, F. and Evan, W.M. (1984) 'Organizational innovation and performance: the problem of organizational lag', *Administrative Science Quarterly*, vol 29, pp 392–409.

Damanpour, F., Walker, M.R. and Avellaneda, N.C. (2009) 'Combinative effects of innovation types and organizational performance: a longitudinal study of service organizations', *Journal of Management Studies*, vol 46, no 4, pp 650–75.

Day, P. and Klein, R. (1987) 'Quality of institutional care and the elderly: policy issues and options', *British Medical Journal*, vol 294, pp 384–7.

Dellot, B. (2014) *Everyday employers*, London: Royal Society for the Arts.

Dellot, B. (2015) *The second age of small*, London: Royal Society for the Arts.

BIS (Department for Business, Innovation and Skills) (2013) *Growing your business: A report on growing micro businesses*, https://www.gov.uk/government/publications/growing-your-business-a-report-on-growing-micro-businesses (accessed 23 August 2013).

Department for Communities and Local Government (2012) *Community right to challenge statutory guidance*, London: Communities and Local Government https://www.gov.uk/government/uploads/system/uploads/attachment_data/file/5990/2168126.pdf (accessed December 2015).

DTI (Department for Trade and Industry) (2002) *Social enterprise: A strategy for success*, London: DTI.

DH (Department of Health) (2005) *Independence, Well-being and Choice*, London: HMSO.

DH (Department of Health) (2006) *Our health, our care, our say: A new direction for community services*, London: HMSO.

DH (2008a) *Social enterprise – Making a difference: A guide to the 'right to request'*, London: Department of Health

DH (2008b) *High quality care for all: NHS next stage review*, The Stationery Office, London.

DH (2009) *Transforming community services: Enabling new patterns of provision*, London: The Stationery Office.

DH (2010) *Supporting micro markets*, London: HMSO.

DH (2011a) *Making quality your business: Guide to the right to provide*, London: Department of Health.

DH (2011b) *Operational guidance to the NHS extending patient choice of provider*, London: Department of Health.

DH (2012) *Caring for our future: Reforming care and support*, London: HMSO

DH (2014) *Care and support statutory guidance issued under the Care Act 2014*, Cabinet Office: London.

DH and NAAPS (2009) *Supporting micromarket development: A concise practical guide for local authorities*, London: Department of Health.

Dickinson, H. (2014) *Performing governance: Partnerships, culture and New Labour*, Basingstoke: Palgrave MacMillan.

Dickinson, H., Allen, K., Alcock, P., Macmillan, R. and Glasby, J. (2012) *The role of the third sector in delivering social care*, London: NIHR School for Social Care Research.

Donahue, K. (2011) 'Have voluntary sector infrastructure support providers failed micro organisations?' *Voluntary Sector Review*, vol 2, no 3, pp 391–8.

Doncaster Council (2011) *Developing new forms of support: Stimulating and supporting the micro social care market*, Doncaster: Doncaster Council.

Downs, A. (1967) *An economic theory of democracy*, New York: Harper and Row.

Duffy, S. (2010) 'The citizenship theory of social justice: exploring the meaning of personalization for social workers', *Journal of Social Work Practice*, vol 24, no 3, pp 253–67.

Duffy, S. (2014) *Unlocking the imagination: Rethinking commissioning* (2nd edn), Sheffield: Centre for Welfare Reform.

Durose, C., Needham, C., Mangan, C. and Rees, J. (2015) 'Generating "good enough" evidence for co-production', *Evidence and Policy*, early view.

Edge, D. (2011) 'Can managed care networks improve perinatal mental healthcare for black and minority ethnic (BME) women?' *Journal of Public Mental Health*, vol 10, no 3, pp 151–63.

Edquist, C., Hommen, L. and McKelvey, M. (2001) *Innovation and employment: Process versus product innovation*, Cheltenham: Edward Elgar Publishing.

Edwards, R. and Alexander, C. (2011) 'Researching with peer/community researchers – ambivalences and tensions', in M. Williams and W.P. Vogt (eds) *The Sage handbook of innovation in social research methods*, London: Sage, pp 269–92.

Edwards, P. and Ram, M. (2006) 'Surviving on the margins of the economy: working relationships in small, low-wage firms', *Journal of Management Studies*, vol 43, no 4, pp 895–916.

Edwards, P., Ram, M. and Black, J. (2004) 'Why does employment legislation not damage small firms?' *Journal of law and society*, vol 31, no 2, pp 245–65.

EHRC (Equality and Human Rights Commission) (2011) *Close to home: An inquiry into older people and human rights in home care*, London: EHRC.

Eldh, A.C., van der Zijpp, T., McMullan, C., McCormack, B., Seers, K. and Rycroft-Malone, J. (2015) '"I have the world's best job" – staff experience of the advantages of caring for older people', *Scandinavian Journal of Caring Services*, DOI: 10.1111/scs.12256.

Ellins, J., Glasby, J., Tanner, D., McIver, S., Davidson, D., Littlechild, R., Snelling, I., Miller, R., Hall, K., Spence, K. and the Care Transitions Project co-researchers (2012) *Understanding and improving transitions of older people: A user and carer centred approach*, London: HMSO/National Institute for Health Research, www.birmingham.ac.uk/documents/news/sdotransitions-report.pdf (accessed 7 April 2016).

Ellis, K. (2015) 'Personalisation, ambiguity and conflict: Matland's model of policy implementation and the "transformation" of adult social care in England', *Policy & Politics*, vol 43, no 2, pp 239–54.

EHRC (Equality and Human Rights Commission) (2011) *Close to home: An inquiry into older people and human rights in home care*, London: EHRC, www.equalityhumanrights.com/publication/close-home-inquiry-older-people-and-human-rights-home-care.

Europa (2003) *The definition of micro, small and medium sized enterprises*, http://europa.eu/legislation_summaries/enterprise/business_environment/n26026_en.htm (accessed 21 August 2013).

Fenwick, T. (2002) 'Transgressive desires: new enterprising selves in the new capitalism', *Work, Employment and Society*, vol 16, no 4, pp 703–23.

Fiedler, B. (2007) *Supporting social care micro providers – A review of the literature*, London: SCIE / NAAPS.

Fielding, J.L. (2008) 'Coding and managing data', in G.N. Gilbert (ed) *Researching social life* (3rd edn), London: Sage, pp 323–52.

Fischer, F. (2003) *Reframing public policy: Discursive politics and deliberative practices*, Oxford: Oxford University Press.

Fischer, F. (2007) 'Policy analysis in critical perspective: the epistemics of discursive practices', *Critical Policy Analysis*, vol 1, no 1, pp 97–109.

Flinders, M., Wood, M. and Cunningham, M. (2015) 'The politics of co-production: risks, limits and pollution', *Evidence and Policy*, early view.

Fox, A. (2013) *Putting people into personalisation: Relational approaches to social care and housing*, Lincoln: ResPublica.

Francis, Lord R. (2012) The Mid Staffordshire NHS Foundation Trust Public Inquiry Chaired by Robert Francis (2012) *Report of the Mid Staffordshire NHS Foundation Trust Public Inquiry (Volumes 1–3)*, London: TSO.

Gaertner, G. and Ramnarayan, S. (1983) 'Organizational effectiveness: an alternative perspective', *Academy of Management Review*, vol 8, pp 97–107.

Gilleard, C. and Higgs, P. (2010) 'Ageing without agency: theorizing the fourth age', *Aging and Mental Health*, vol 14, no 2, pp 121–8.

Glasby, J. and Dickinson, H. (2009) (eds) *International perspectives on health and social care*, Oxford: Wiley-Blackwell.

Glasby, J. and Littlechild, R. (2016) *Direct payments and personal budgets: Putting personalisation into practice* (3rd edn), Bristol: The Policy Press.

Glendinning, C., Challis, D., Fernandez, J.-L., Jacobs, S., Jones, K., Knapp, M., Manthorpe, J., Moran, N., Netten, A., Stevens, M. and Wilberforce, M. (2008) *Evaluation of the Individual Budgets pilot programme*, Final report, Social Policy Research Unit, University of York.

Goffman, E. (1968) *Asylums*, Harmondsworth: Pelican.

Gordon, C. (1991) 'Governmental rationality: an introduction', in G. Burchell, C. Gordon and P. Miller (eds) *The Foucault effect: Studies in governmental rationality*, London: Harvester Wheatsheaf, pp 1–52.

Gould, S.J. (1988) *Time's arrow, time's cycle*, Harmondsworth: Penguin.

Gray, A.M. and Birrell, D. (2013) *Transforming adult social care: Contemporary policy and practice*, Bristol: The Policy Press.

Gray, A. and Jenkins, B. (2011) 'Policy evaluation: many powers, many truths', in F. Eliadis, J. Furubo and S. Jacob (eds) *Evaluation: Seeking truth or power?* New Brunswick/London: Transaction Publishers.

Gray, B.H., Sarnak, D.O. and Burgers, J.S. (2015) *Home care by self-governing nurse teams: The Netherlands Buurtzorg model*, New York: The Commonwealth Fund.

Greenhalgh, T. and Peacock, R. (2005) 'Effectiveness and efficiency of search methods in systematic reviews of complex evidence: audit of primary sources', *British Medical Journal*, vol 331, no 7524, p 1064.

Greenhalgh, T., Russell, J. and Swinglehurst, D. (2005) 'Narrative methods in quality improvement research', *BMJ Quality and Safety*, vol 14, pp 443–9.

Greenhalgh, T., Robert, G., Bate, P., Kyriakidou, O., Macfarlane, F. and Peacock, R. (2004) *How to spread good ideas: A systematic review of the literature on diffusion, dissemination and sustainability of innovations in health service delivery and organisation*, London: National Institute for Health Research.

Grit, K. and de Bont, A (2010) 'Tailor-made finance versus tailor-made care. Can the state strengthen consumer choice in health care by reforming the financial structure of long-term care?' *Journal of Medical Ethics*, vol 36, no 2, pp 79-83.

Hajer, M. (2006) 'Doing discourse analysis: coalitions, practices, meaning', in M. van den Brink and T. Metze (eds) *Words matter in policy and planning: Discourse theory and method in the social sciences*, Utrecht, KNAG/Nethur: Netherlands Geographical Studies, vol 344, pp 65–74.

Hall, K., Alcock, P. and Millar, R. (2012a) 'Start up and sustainability: marketisation and the social enterprise investment fund in England', *Journal of Social Policy*, vol 41, no 4, pp 733–49.

Hall, K., Miller, R. and Millar, R. (2012b) 'Jumped or pushed: what motivates NHS staff to set up a social enterprise?' *Social Enterprise Journal*, vol 8, no 1, pp 49–62.

Hardill, I. and Dwyer, P. (2011) 'Delivering public services in the mixed economy of welfare: perspectives from the voluntary and community sector in rural England', *Journal of Social Policy*, vol 40, no 1, pp 157–72.

Harris, M. and Albury, D. (2009) *The innovation imperative*, London: NESTA, www.nesta.org.uk/the-innovation-imperative/ (accessed November 2015).

Harrison, B. (1997) *Lean and mean: Why large corporations will continue to dominate the global economy*, New York: Guilford Press.

Hatch, M.J. and Schultz, M. (1997) 'Relations between organizational culture, identity and image', *European Journal of Marketing*, vol 31, no 5–6, pp 356–65.

Haveman, H.A. (2003) 'Organisational size and change: diversification in the savings and loan industry after deregulation', *Administrative Science Quarterly*, vol 38, pp 20–50.

Hazenberg, R. and Hall, K. (2014) 'Public service mutuals: towards a theoretical understanding of the spin-out process', *Policy and Politics*, DOI 10.1332/147084414X13988685244243.

Henwood, M. (2010) *Journeys without maps: The decisions and destinations of people who self-fund – a qualitative study from Melanie Henwood Associates*, London: Putting People First.

Henwood, M. (2014) 'Self-funders: the road from perdition?' in C. Needham and J. Glasby (eds) *Debates in personalisation*, Bristol: The Policy Press.

HM Government (2008) *Carers at the heart of 21stcentury families and communities*, London: HMSO.

HM Government (2010) *The Coalition: Our programme for government*, https://www.gov.uk/government/news/the-coalition-our-programme-for-government (accessed 12 May 2015).

HM Government (2015) *Setting up a social enterprise*, https://www.gov.uk/set-up-a-social-enterprise (accessed 26 November 2015).

Higgs, P. and Gilleard, C. (2015) *Rethinking old age: Theorizing the fourth age*, London: Palgrave Macmillan.

Hill, C.J. and Lynn, L.E. (2005) 'Is hierarchical governance in decline? Evidence from empirical research', *Journal of Public Administration Research and Theory*, vol 15, no 2, pp 173–95.

Hitt, M A., Hoskisson, R.E. and Hicheon, K. (1997) 'International diversification: on innovation and firm performance in product-diversified firms', *Academy of Management Journal*, vol 40, pp 767–98.

Holman, B. (1996) 'Fifty years ago: the Curtis and Clyde reports', *Children and Society*, vol 10, pp 197–209.

Hood, C. (1991) 'A public management for all seasons', *Public Administration*, vol 69, no 1, pp 3–19.

House of Lords (2013) *Ready for ageing? Report of the select committee on public service and demographic change*, Session 2012–13, www. publications.parliament.uk/pa/ld201213/ldselect/ldpublic/140/140. pdf.

HSCIC (2015) *Personal social services: Expenditure and unit costs England 2014–15: Final release*, www.hscic.gov.uk/catalogue/PUB19165/ pss-exp-eng-14–15-fin-rep.pdf.

In Control (no date a) 'What is self-directed support?', www.in-control. org.uk/support/support-for-individuals,-family-members-carers/ what-is-self-directed-support.aspx (accessed 6 April 2016).

In Control (no date b) 'Shop for support', https://www.shop4support. com/s4s/CustomPage/Index/62 (accessed 6 April 2016).

INVOLVE (2013) *Exploring the impact of public involvement on the quality of research*, Eastleigh: INVOLVE.

IPC (Institute of Public Care) (2011) *People who pay for care: An analysis of self-funders in the social care market*, Oxford: Oxford Brookes University.

Izuhara, M. (2003) 'Social Inequality under a New Social Contract: Long-term care in Japan, *Social Policy and Administration*, vol 37, no 4, pp 395–410.

Jeffares, S. (2014) *Interpretive hashtag politics: Policy ideas in an era of social media*, Basingstoke: Palgrave Macmillan.

Joseph, K. (1975) *Reversing the trend: A critical re-appraisal of conservative economic and social policies: seven speeches*, Chichester: Rose.

Kelly, P. (2006) 'The entrepreneurial self and "youth at-risk": exploring the horizons of identity in the twenty-first century', *Journal of Youth Studies*, vol 9, no 1, pp 17–32.

Kirkpatrick, I. (2006) 'Between markets and networks: the reform of social care provision in the UK', *Revista de Analisis Economico*, vol 21, no 2, pp 43–59.

Kooiman, J. (2003) *Governing as governance*, London: Sage.

Kotecha, N. (2009) 'Black and minority ethnic women', in S. Fernando and F. Keating (eds) *Mental health in a multi-ethnic society: A multidisciplinary handbook* (2nd edn), London: Routledge.

Laloux, F. (2014) *Reinventing organizations: A guide to creating organizations inspired by the next stage of human consciousness*, Belgium: Nelson Parker.

Land, H. and Himmelweit, S. (2010) *Who cares, who pays? A report on personalisation in social care prepared by UNISON*, London: UNISON.

Leadbeater, C. (2004) *Personalization through participation: A new script for public services*, London: Demos.

Leat, D. (2003) *Replicating successful voluntary sector projects*, London: Association of Charitable Foundations, http://baringfoundation.org.uk/wp-content/uploads/2014/10/ACFRepReport6.pdf.

Leece, J. (2010) 'Paying the piper and calling the tune: power and the direct payment relationship' *British Journal of Social Work*, vol 40, no 1, pp 188–206.

Leece, J. and Peace, S. (2010) 'Developing new understandings of independence and autonomy in the personalised relationship', *British Journal of Social Work*, vol 40, no 6, pp 1847–65.

Leonard Cheshire Disability (2013) *Ending 15 minute care*, London: Leonard Cheshire Disability. www.leonardcheshire.org/sites/default/files/15%20min%20care%20report%20final.pdf.

Lewis, J. and Meredith, B. (1989) *Daughters who care*, London: Routledge.

Lewis, J. and West, A. (2014) 'Re-shaping social care services for older people in England: policy development and the problem of achieving "Good Care"', *Journal of Social Policy*, vol 43, pp 1–18.

LGA (Local Government Association) (2015) *Commissioning for better outcomes: A route map*, London: Local Government Association, www.local.gov.uk/documents/10180/5756320/Commissioning+for+Better+Outcomes+A+route+map/8f18c36f-805c-4d5e-b1f5-d3755394cfab.

LGA/Locality (2012) *Empowering Communities*, London: LGA, http://locality.org.uk/wp-content/uploads/Empowering-communities-making-the-most-of-local-assets-a-councillors-guide.pdf

Littlechild, R. and Tanner, D. (2015) *Does smaller mean better? Evaluating micro-enterprises in adult social care: Evaluation of co-researcher involvement*, Birmingham: University of Birmingham www.birmingham.ac.uk/Documents/college-social-sciences/social-policy/HSMC/rescarch/micro-enterprise/evaluation-of-co-researcher-involvement.pdf (accessed 6 April 2016).

Lloyd, L. (2010) 'The individual in social care: the ethics of care and the "personalisation agenda" in services for older people in England', *Ethics and Social Welfare*, vol 4, no 2, pp 188–200.

Lloyd, L. (2012) *Health and care in ageing societies: A new international approach*, Bristol: The Policy Press.

Lloyd, L. (2014) 'Can personalisation work for older people?', in C. Needham and J. Glasby (eds) *Debates in personalisation*, Bristol: The Policy Press, pp 55–64.

Locality (2014) *Saving money by doing the right thing*, London: Locality, http://locality.org.uk/wp-content/uploads/Locality-Report-Diseconomies-web-version.pdf (accessed 15 May 2015).

Lockwood, S. (2013) 'Community assets helping to deliver health and well-being and tackle health inequalities', *Journal of Integrated Care*, vol 21, no 1, pp 26–33.

Lyon, F. and Fernandez, H. (2012) *Scaling up social enterprise: Strategies taken from early years providers*, TSRC Working Paper 79, Birmingham: Third Sector Research Centre.

Lyotard, J. (1984) *The postmodern condition: A report on knowledge development*, Manchester: Manchester University Press.

McCabe, A. and Phillimore, J. (2012) *All change? Surviving 'below the radar': community groups and activities in a Big Society*, TSRC Working Paper 87, Birmingham: Third Sector Research Centre.

McCabe, A., Phillimore, J. and Mayblin, L. (2010) *'Below the radar' activities and organisations in the third sector: A summary review of the literature*, Briefing paper 29, Birmingham: Third Sector Research Centre.

MacGillivray, A., Conaty, P. and Wadhams, C. (2001) *Low flying heroes: Micro social enterprise below the radar screen*, London: New Economics Foundation.

McKay, S., Moro, D., Teasdale, S. and Clifford, D. (2011) *The marketisation of charities in England and Wales*, TSRC Working Paper 69, Birmingham: Third Sector Research Centre.

McLaughlin, H. (2009) 'Keeping service user involvement in research honest', *British Journal of Social work*, 40: 1591–1608.

Macmillan, R. (2011) *Seeing things differently? The promise of qualitative longitudinal research on the third sector*, TSRC Working Paper 56, Birmingham: Third Sector Research Centre.

Macmillan, R. (2012) *'Distinction' in the third sector*, TSRC Working Paper 89, Birmingham: Third Sector Research Centre.

Macmillan, R. (2013) '"Distinction" in the third sector', *Voluntary Sector Review*, vol 4, no 1, pp 39–54.

Macmillan, R., Taylor, R., Arvidson, M., Soteri-Proctor, A. and Teasdale, S. (2013) *The third sector in unsettled times: A field guide*, TSRC Working Paper 109, Birmingham, Third Sector Research Centre.

Major, D. (2011) *What do we mean by scale?* Washington, DC: Grantmakers for Effective Organisations.

Mallett, O. and Wapshott, R. (2015) 'Making sense of self employment in late career: understanding the identity work of olderpreneurs', *Work, Employment and Society*, vol 29, no 2, pp 250– 266.

Matlay, H. (1999) 'Employee relations in small firms: a micro-business perspective', *Employee Relations*, vol 21, no 3, pp 285–95.

Maynard-Moody, S. and Musheno, H. (2003) *Cops, teachers, counselors: Stories from the front lines of public service*, Ann Arbor: University of Michigan Press.

Mazzucato, M. (2013) *The entrepreneurial state: Debunking public vs. private myths in risk and innovation*, London: Anthem Press.

McLaughlin, H. (2009) 'Keeping service user involvement in research honest', *British Journal of Social work*, 40:1591–1608

Mencap (2012) *Stuck at home: The impact of day service cuts on people with a learning disability*, London: Mencap.

Miles, M.B., Huberman, A.M. and Saldaña, J. (2014) *Qualitative data analysis: A methods sourcebook* (3rd edn), London: Sage.

Miller, R. and Lyon, F. (2016) 'Spinning with substance? The creation of new third sector organisations from public services', in J. Rees and D. Mullins (eds) *The third sector in public services: Developments, innovations and challenges*, Bristol: The Policy Press.

Milligan, C. (2009) *There's no place like home: Place and care in an ageing society*, London: Ashgate.

Mohan, J., Kane, D., Wilding, K., Branson, J. and Owles, F. (2010) 'Beyond "flat-earth" maps of the third sector: enhancing our understanding of the contribution of "below-radar" organisations', *Third sector trends study*, Newcastle-upon-Tyne: Northern Rock Foundation.

Mol, A. (2008) *The logic of care: Health and the problem of patient choice*, London: Routledge.

Mueller, D.C. (1972) 'A life cycle theory of the firm', *The Journal of Industrial Economics*, vol 20, no 3, pp 199–219.

Mulgan, G. (2007) *Social innovation: What is it, why it matters and how it can be accelerated*, London: The Young Foundation.

NAAPS (National Association of Adult Placement Schemes) (2008) *Micro markets project: Report on progress after one year*, London: NAAPS.

NAAPS (2010) *Cuts or putting people first*, London: National Association of Adult Placement Schemes.

National Audit Office (2010) *Progress in improving stroke care*, London: The Stationery Office, https://www.nao.org.uk/wp-content/uploads/2010/02/0910291.pdf.

NAVCA (2013) *Social value*, London: NAVCA, www.navca.org.uk/socialvalue (accessed 15 May 2014).

NCVO (National Council for Voluntary Organisations) (2011) *Counting the cuts: The impact of spending cuts on the UK voluntary and community sector*, https://www.ncvo.org.uk/images/documents/policy_and_research/funding/counting_the_cuts_2013.pdf.

NCVO (2015) *UK civil society almanac 2015*, London: NCVO.

NDTI (National Development Team for Inclusion) (2013) *Co-production involving and led by older people*, www.ndti.org.uk/uploads/files/Coproductionandolderpeople.pdf (accessed 26 November 2015).

NDTI and Helen Sanderson Associates (2010) *Personalisation: Don't just do it, coproduce it and live it! A guide to coproduction with older people*, Stockport: HAS Press.

Needham, C. (2003) *Citizen-consumers: New Labour's marketplace democracy*, London: Catalyst.

Needham, C. (2007) *The reform of public services under New Labour: Narratives of consumerism*, Basingstoke: Palgrave Macmillan.

Needham, C. (2011) *Personalising public services: Understanding the personalisation narrative*, Bristol: The Policy Press.

Needham, C. (2014) 'Personalisation: from day centres to community hubs?' *Critical Social Policy*, vol 34, no 1, pp 47–65.

Needham, C. (2015) 'The spaces of personalisation: place and distance in caring labour', *Social Policy and Society*, vol 14, no 3, pp 357–69.

Needham, C. and Carr, S. (2009) *Co-production and social care*, London: Social Care Institute for Excellence.

Needham, C. and Carr, S. (2015) 'Micro-provision of social care support for marginalised communities: filling the gap or building bridges to the mainstream?' *Social Policy and Administration*, DOI: 10.1111/spol.12114.

Needham, C. and Glasby, J. (eds) (2014) *Debates in personalisation*, Bristol: The Policy Press.

Needham, C. and Tizard, J. (2010) *Commissioning for personalisation: From the fringes to the mainstream*, London: Chartered Institute of Public Finance and Accountancy/Public Management and Policy Association.

Netten, A., Jones, K. and Sandhu, S. (2007) 'Provider and care workforce influences on quality of home-care services in England', *Journal of Aging and Social Policy*, vol 19, no 3, pp 81–97.

NHS (2014) *Five year forward view*, London: Department of Health, https://www.england.nhs.uk/wp-content/uploads/2014/10/5yfv-web.pdf (accessed 7 April 2016).

NHS Confederation (2012) *Working locally: Micro-enterprises and building community assets*, Working Paper 4, May 2012, London: NHS Confederation.

NHS England (2015) *NHS launches new collaboration to sustain and improve local hospitals*, https://www.england.nhs.uk/2015/05/20/improving-local-hospitals/.

NHS Foundation (2011) *NHS Fife: Micro-enterprise care solutions to reduce acute hospital admissions*, www.health.org.uk/areas-of-work/programmes/shine-eleven/related-projects/nhs-fife/.

NICE (National Institute for Health and Care Excellence) (2015) *Home care: Delivering personal care and 10 practical support to older people living in 11 their own homes*, Draft Guidance, www.nice.org.uk/guidance/gid-scwave0713/documents/home-care-draft-full-guideline2.

NIHR (2013) *Budgeting for involvement: Practical advice on budgeting for actively involving the public in research studies*, MHRN and INVOLVE, www.invo.org.uk/wp-content/uploads/2014/11/10002-INVOLVE-Budgeting-Tool-Publication-WEB.pdf (accessed 16 December 2015).

Niskanen, W.A. (1971) *Bureaucracy and representative government*, Chicago: Aldine Atherton.

O'Mahoney, J. and Vincent, S. (2014) 'Critical realism as an empirical project', in P.K. Edwards, J. O'Mahoney and S. Vincent (eds) *Studying organizations using critical realism*, Oxford: Oxford University Press, pp 1–20.

Omachonu, V.K. and Einspruch, N.G. (2010) 'Innovation in healthcare delivery systems: a conceptual framework', *The Innovation Journal: The Public Sector Innovation Journal*, vol 15, no 1, pp 2–20.

Osborne, S.P. (ed) (2010) *The new public governance: Emerging perspectives on the theory and practice of public governance*, London: Routledge.

Panitch, L. and Leys, C. (2001) *The end of parliamentary socialism: From New Left to New Labour* (2nd edn), London: Verso.

Pattie, C. and Johnston, R. (2011) 'How big is the big society?' *Parliamentary Affairs*, vol 64, no 3, pp 403–24.

Pawson, R. and Tilley, N. (1997) *Realistic evaluation*, London: Sage.

Pearson, S.D. and Rawlins, M.D. (2005) 'Quality, innovation, and value for money: NICE and the British National Health Service', *Journal of the American Medical Association*, vol 294, no 20, pp 2618–22.

Pearson, C., Ridley, J. and Hunter, S. (2014) *Self-directed support: Personalisation, choice and control*, Edinburgh: Dunedin Press.

Peck, E. and Dickinson, H. (2009) *Performing leadership*, Basingstoke: Palgrave Macmillan.

Peckham, S., Exworthy, M., Powell, M. and Greener, I. (2005) *Decentralisation, centralisation and devolution in publicly funded health services: Decentralisation as an organisational model for health care in England*, Report for the National Co-ordinating Centre for NHS Service Delivery and Organization R&D (NCCSDO).

Phillimore, J., McCabe, A. and Soteri-Proctor, A. (2009) *Under the radar? Researching unregistered and informal third sector activity*, Birmingham: University of Birmingham.

Poll, C. (2007) 'Co-production in supported housing: KeyRing living support networks and neighbourhood networks', *Research Highlights in Social Work: Co-Production and Personalisation in Social Care Changing Relationships in the Provision of Social Care*, vol 49, pp 49–66.

Pollitt, C. (2003) 'Theoretical overview', in C. Pollitt and C. Talbot (eds) *Unbundled government: A critical analysis of the global trend to agencies, quangos and contractualisation*, London: Routledge, pp 319–41.

Pollitt, C. (2008) *Time, policy, management: Governing with the past*, Oxford: Oxford University Press.

Popay, J., Rogers, A. and Williams, G. (1998) 'Rationale and standards for the systematic review of qualitative literature in health services research', *Qualitative Health Research*, vol 8, no 3, pp 341–51.

Postma, J. (2015) 'Scaling care', PhD thesis, Rotterdam: Erasmus University.

Powell, M. (2007) *Understanding the mixed economy of welfare*, Bristol: The Policy Press.

Powell, W.W. and DiMaggio, P.J. (eds) (2012) *The new institutionalism in organizational analysis*, Chicago: University of Chicago Press.

PSSRU (Personal Social Services Research Unit) (2010) *Unit costs of health and social care*, Canterbury: University of Kent, Personal Social Services Research Unit. www.pssru.ac.uk/pdf/uc/uc2010/uc2010. pdf.

Public Accounts Committee (2011) *Oversight of user choice and provider competition in care markets*, 57th report, London: The Stationery Office, http://www.publications.parliament.uk/pa/cm201012/cmselect/cmpubacc/1530/1530.pdf

Public Accounts Committee (2015) *Care Quality Commission, 12th report, London: The Stationery Office, http://www.publications.parliament. uk/pa/cm201516/cmselect/cmpubacc/501/501.pdf*

Putting People First (2007) *Putting people first: A shared vision and commitment to the transformation of adult social care*, London: HM Government.

Quinn, J.B. (1985) 'Managing innovation: controlled chaos', *Harvard Business Review*, May–June, pp 75–84.

Rainey, G. and Steinbauer, P. (1999) 'Galloping elephants: developing elements of a theory of effective government organizations', *Journal of Public Administration Research and Theory*, vol 9, no 1, pp 1–32.

Ram, M and Jones, T (2008) *Ethnic Minorities in Business*, Milton Keynes: Small Business Research Trust.

Ram, M. and Trehan, K. (2010) 'Critical action learning, policy learning and small firms: an inquiry', *Management Learning*, vol 41, no 4, pp 415–28.

Rees, J. (2014) 'Public sector commissioning and the third sector: old wine in new bottles?' *Public Policy and Administration*, DOI: 10.1177/0952076713510345.

Rees, J. and Mullins, D. (eds) (2016) *The third sector in public services: Developments, innovations and challenges*, Bristol: The Policy Press.

Rees, J., Mullins, D. and Bovaird, T. (2012) *Third sector partnerships for public service delivery: An evidence review*, TSRC Working Paper 60, Birmingham: Third Sector Research Centre.

Rhodes, R.A.W. (1997) *Understanding governance: Policy networks, governance, reflexivity and accountability*, Buckingham: Open University Press.

Riessman, C. (1993) *Narrative analysis* (Qualitative research methods series 30), London: Sage.

Riessman, C. (2001) 'Analysis of personal narratives', in J.F. Gubrium and J.A. Holstein (eds) *Handbook of interviewing*, London: Sage.

Roulstone, A. and Morgan, H. (2009) 'Neo-liberal individualism or self-directed support: are we all speaking the same language on modernising adult social care?' *Social Policy and Society*, vol 8, no 3, pp 333–45.

Roy, A. (2012) 'Avoiding the involvement overdose: drugs, race, ethnicity and participatory research practice', *Critical Social Policy*, vol 32, pp 636–54.

Samuel, M. (2013) *Expert guide to direct payments, personal budgets and individual budgets*, www.communitycare.co.uk/articles/30/01/2013/102669/direct-paymentspersonal-budgets-and-individual-budgets.htm (accessed 6 April 2016).

Sawbridge, Y. and Needham, C. (2014) 'Emotionally qualified', *Nursing Standard*, vol 29, no 13, pp 26–7.

Sayer, A. (2000) *Realism and social science*, London: Sage.

Scherer, F.M. and Ross, D. (1990) *Industrial market structure and economic performance*, Boston, MA: Houghton Mifflin.

Schilling, M.A. and Steensma, H.K. (2001) 'The use of modular organizational forms: an industry-level analysis', *Academy of Management Journal*, vol 44, no 6, pp 1149–68.

Schumpeter, J. (1934) *The theory of economic development*, Cambridge, MA: Harvard University Press.

Schwartz-Shea, P. and Yanow, D. (2012) *Interpretive approaches to research design: Concepts and processes*, New York: Routledge.

SCIE (2010) *At a glance 29: Personalisation briefing – Implications for social workers in adults' services*, London: SCIE, www.scie.org.uk/publications/ataglance/ataglance29.asp.

SCIE (2012) *Report 61: Co-production and participation: Older people with high support needs*, www.scie.org.uk/publications/reports/report61/ (accessed 26 November 2015).

Scourfield, P. (2004) 'Questions raised for local authorities when old people are evicted from their care homes', *British Journal of Social Work*, vol 34, no 4, pp 501–16.

Scourfield, P. (2006) 'What matters is what works? How discourses of modernisation have both silenced and limited debate on domiciliary care for older people', *Critical Social Policy*, vol 25, no 5, pp 5–30.

Scourfield, P. (2007) 'Social care and the modern citizen: client, consumer, service user, manager and entrepreneur', *British Journal of Social Work*, vol 37, pp 107–22.

SEUK (2012) *The social value guide: Implementing the Public Services (Social Value) Act*, www.socialenterprise.org.uk/uploads/files/2012/12/social_value_guide.pdf (accessed December 2015).

Shared Lives Plus (no date) *Shared lives, micro-enterprise and Homeshare: Supporting older people*, Liverpool: Shared Lives Plus.

Shared Lives Plus (2011) *Briefing: Research and evaluation opportunities*, http://sharedlivesplus.org.uk/images/publications/SLPlus-research-briefing-Jan-13.pdf (accessed 12 August 2015).

Sheaff, R., Schofield, J., Mannion, R., Dowling, B., Marshall, M. and McNally, R. (2004) *Organisational factors and performance: A review*, Report for the NCCSDO.

Silverman, D. (2013) *Doing qualitative research* (4th edn), London: Sage.

Sin, C.H. (2006) 'Expectations of support among White British and Asian-Indian older people in Britain: the interdependence of formal and informal spheres', *Health and Social Care in the Community*, vol 14, no 3, pp 215–24.

Skelcher, C. (2008) 'Does governance perform? Concepts, evidence, causalities and research strategies', in J. Hartley, C. Donaldson, C. Skelcher and M. Wallace (eds) *Managing to improve public services*, Cambridge: Cambridge University Press, pp 27–45.

Skills for Care (2013) *The size and structure of the adult social care sector and workforce in England 2013* (September), Leeds: Skills for Care.

Skills for Care (2015) *The state of the adult social care sector and workforce in England*, London: Skills for Care, www.skillsforcare.org.uk/Document-library/NMDS-SC,-workforce-intelligence-and-innovation/NMDS-SC/State-of-2014-ENGLAND-WEB-FINAL.pdf#page=4.

Slasberg, C., Beresford, P. and Schofield, P. (2012a) 'How self-directed support is failing to deliver personal budgets and personalisation', *Research, Policy and Planning*, vol 29, no 3, pp 161–77.

Slasberg, C., Beresford, P. and Schofield, P. (2012b) 'Can personal budgets really deliver better outcome for all at no cost? Reviewing the evidence, costs and quality', *Disability and Society*, vol 27, no 7, pp 1029–34.

Smith, J., Holder, H., Edwards, N., Maybin, J., Parker, H., Rosen, R. and Walsh, N. (2013) *Securing the future of general practice: New models of primary care*, London: Kings Fund/Nuffield Trust, www. humbersidelmc.org.uk/uploads/3/7/5/8/37582639/130718_ securing_the_future_of_general_practice-_full_report_0.pdf (accessed 15 June 2015).

Social Enterprise Academy (2013) *Micro-enterprise: Turning ideas into reality*, www.socialcareideasfactory.com/files/2513/7277/1094/ Social_Care_Ideas_Factory_2013.pdf (accessed 23 August 2013).

Spandler, H. (2004) 'Friend or foe? Towards a critical assessment of direct payments', *Critical Social Policy*, vol 24, no 2, pp 187–209.

Steckley, L. (2015) 'Care ethics and physical restraint in residential child care', in M. Barnes, T. Brannelly, L. Ward and N. Ward (eds) *Ethics of care: Critical advances in international perspective*, Bristol: The Policy Press, pp 195–206.

Storey, D. (1994) *Understanding the small business sector*, London: Routledge.

Talbot, C. (2010) *Theories of performance: Organizational and service improvement in the public domain*, Oxford: Oxford University Press.

Talbot, C. and Johnson, C. (2006) 'Big is beautiful (again)', *Public Finance*, 6 January, www.publicfinance.co.uk/2006/01/big-beautiful-again-colin-talbot-and-carole-johnson (accessed 12 May 2014).

Tanner, D. (2017) 'Co-research and communicative action: what does it contribute?', forthcoming.

Teasdale, S. (2011) 'What's in a name? Making sense of social enterprise discourses', *Public Policy and Administration*, vol 27, no 2, pp 99–119.

Teasdale, S., Lyon, F. and Baldock, R. (2013) 'Playing with numbers: a methodological critique of the social enterprise growth myth', *Journal of Social Entrepreneurship*, vol 4, no 2, pp 113–31.

Teisman, G. and Klijn, E.H. (2008) 'Complexity theory and public management', *Public Management Review*, vol 10, no 3, pp 287–97.

TLAP (Think Local, Act Personal) *Peer support and the personalisation of adult social care*, London: TLAP, http://www.thinklocalactpersonal. org.uk/Latest/Peer-support-and-the-personalisation-of-adult-social-care/

TLAP (2011) *Developing social care micro markets*, www. thinklocalactpersonal.org.uk/Regions/EastMidlands/CMD/MicroMarkets/ (accessed November 2015).

Tsoukas, H. and Chia, R. (2002) 'On organizational becoming: rethinking organizational change', *Organization Science*, vol 13, pp 567–82.

Tunstill, J. and Blewitt, J. (2013) 'Mapping the journey: outcome focused practice and the role of interim outcomes in family support services', *Child and Family Social Work*, vol 20, no 2, pp 234–43.

Twigg, J. (2000) 'Carework as a form of bodywork', *Ageing and Society*, vol 20, no 4, pp 389–411.

Ungerson, C. (1983) 'Why do women care?', in J. Finch and D. Groves (eds) *A labour of love: Women, work and caring*, London: Routledge and Kegan Paul, pp 31–40.

Ungerson, C. (1987) *Policy is personal: Sex, gender and informal care*, London: Tavistock.

UNISON (2014) '15 minute home care visits in England on the rise', www.unison.org.uk/content/conNewsArticle/5637 (accessed 24 April 2015).

Valios, N. (2007) 'What must smaller charities do to gain public sector contracts?', *Community Care*, 12 April, pp 16–17.

Van de Venn, A.H. and Rogers, E.M. (1988) 'Innovation and organizations: critical perspectives', *Communication Research*, vol 15, pp 632–51.

Veblen, T. (1970) *The theory of the leisure class*, London: Unwin.

Wagenaar, M. (2011) *Meaning in action*, New York: M.E. Sharpe.

Wainwright, H. (1994) *Arguments for a new Left: Answering the free-market Right*, Oxford: Blackwell.

Waldrop, M. (1994) *Complexity: The emerging science at the edge of order and chaos*, London: Penguin.

Walker R.M. (2008) 'An empirical evaluation of innovation types and organizational and environmental characteristics: towards a configuration framework', *Journal of Public Administration Research and Theory*, vol 18, pp 591–615.

Walker, R.M. (2014) 'Internal and external antecedents of process innovation: a review and extension', *Public Management Review*, vol 16, no 1, pp 21–44.

Walsh, K. and Shutes, I. (2013) 'Care relationships, quality of care and migrant 13 workers caring for older people', *Ageing and Society*, vol 33, pp 393–420.

Wanless, D. (2006) *Securing good care for older people: Taking a long term view*, London: King's Fund.

Ward, N. (2015) 'Reciprocity and mutuality: people with learning disabilities as carers', in M. Barnes, T. Brannelly, L. Ward and N. Ward (eds) *Ethics of care: Critical advances in international perspective*, Bristol: The Policy Press, pp 165–78.

Watson, T.J. (2009) 'Entrepreneurial action, identity work and the use of multiple discursive resources: the case of a rapidly changing family business', *International Small Business Journal*, vol 27, no 3, pp 251–74.

Weber, M. (1997) 'Rational legal authority and bureaucracy', in M. Hill (ed) *The policy process: A reader*, London: Prentice Hall, pp 323–7.

Webb, S. and Webb, B. (1920) *A constitution for the socialist commonwealth of Great Britain*, London: Longmans, Green and Co.

Weick, K. (1988) 'Enacted sensemaking in crisis situations', *Journal of Management Studies*, vol 25, pp 305–17.

Wengraf, T. (2001) *Qualitative interviewing: Biographic narrative and semi-structured methods*, London: Sage Publications.

West, K. (2013) 'The grip of personalization in adult social care: between managerial domination and fantasy', *Critical Social Policy*, vol 33, no 4, pp 638–57.

Williams, C. (2003) 'Developing community involvement: contrasting local and regional participatory cultures in Britain and their implications for policy', *Regional Studies*, vol 37, pp 531–42.

Williams, R. (2010) 'Innovation', in R. Ashworth, G. Boyne and T. Entwistle (eds) *Public service improvement: Theories and evidence*, Oxford: Oxford University Press, pp 143–61.

Yanow, D. (2007) 'Interpretation in policy analysis: on methods and practice', *Critical Policy Analysis*, vol 1, no 1, pp 110–22.

Yeandle, S. and Stiell, B. (2007) 'Issues in the development of the direct payments scheme for older people in England', in C. Ungerson and S. Yeandle (eds) *Cash for care in developed welfare states*, Basingstoke, Hampshire: Palgrave.

Young, D. (2001) 'Organizational identity in nonprofit organizations: strategic and structural implications', *Nonprofit, management and leadership*, vol 12, no 2, pp 139–57.

Index

Printed and bound by CPI Group (UK) Ltd, Croydon, CR0 4YY

27/10/2024

14580557-0004